Juicing Joy: With Fruits, Berries And Melons

By Oran Kangas

Table of Contents

Preface

The many health advantages available through juicing all start from one simple truth:

Vegetables, fruits, and other organic foods provide great nutrition, yet even that can be massively increased.

This occurs by means of a special machine designed to:

- Take in healthy organic materials.
- Extract every last drop of nutrients available.
- Expel the difficult to digest debris.
- And deliver the results as a liquid.

Called juicing, this process of transformation turns veggies from a good idea into a great one.

Juicing nourishes your system with life-giving enzymes and whole, unprocessed nutrients. Some your body has been missing ... for months.

To maximize those precious enzymes, consume the juice the instant it's produced.

21 Days To A Healthy Lifestyle

It takes at least 21 days for the average individual to form a new habit. If you would make juicing your healthy healing habit, it is imperative that you make a 21 day commitment to incorporate juicing into your life.

That will get you started.

What will keep you coming back, year after year, is that it is beyond healthy it is actually a totally new way to eat a culinary lifestyle that is delicious, nutritious, fast, and easy.

Meanwhile, your body will do something unexpected. It will heal itself ... from the inside out.

How? you wonder. Well, that is what this whole book is about.

But here is a 1 paragraph summary:

A juicing machine extracts the maximum nutrients from healthy fruits and vegetables. It delivers them in the easiest form to digest liquid. So you get MORE healthy NUTRITION in the healthiest possible FORM.

It's no wonder that the health benefits claimed by users border on the unbelievable.

Let's examine a few such claims from people who have gone from reading to action.

12 Big Picture Health Benefits Of Fresh Juicing

This is why you might consider a 21 day commitment.

Reason #1: the first system in your body where you will likely notice healing is digestion. Among the ingredients available to you will be critical enzymes for optimal assimilation of food. The juiced form of nutrients will enter your stomach already broken down, so they can quickly pass through without taxing the digestive system ... for the first time in years.

Reason #2: without exercising, you can effortlessly lose weight. With your body suddenly getting what it needs, your cravings are eliminated.

Reason #3: your body will have increased energy, more than it has felt in years. This huge influx of concentrated nutrients comes pouring in: finding, binding, sealing, healing, procuring, curing, everything, everywhere.

Its liquid energy, pre-digested form does not require energy to digest, it creates new energy.

Reason #4: the body will seek to redistribute that new-found energy to heal its tired, abused self. Like arid, parched earth, parts of the body will absorb energy faster than others. Perhaps it is handling an ulcer, dealing with arthritis pain, or unclogging arteries. Soon sated, the energy will flow on, seeking out new aches and pains to soothe.

Reason #5: you will be eating healthier food products than ever before. More nutrients, less toxins, more positive chemical activity within your body, and a massive influx of pure nutrition that your body has never before experienced.

Reason #6: Then your immune system (with its new-found riches of antioxidants, vitamins, energy and nutrients) will kick in, to produce increased over-all health. The strengthened immune system will seek and destroy any new threats it finds – perhaps a tumor will be stopped in its tracks.

Reason #7: The immune system will empower local systems to switch from defense to offense in dealing with internal problems. Even externally, the skin will begin to tighten and improve.

Reason #8: Cell repair and regeneration will allow your body will begin healing old wounds. Current problems will start to get better, engulfed in life-giving blood and healing micro-nutrients. Whatever has been lacking at the cellular level is suddenly present.

Reason #9: Your entire body-system will begin to detoxify naturally as less toxins are being thrust into your body, plus the body itself will begin to fight back aggressively to eliminate toxic accumulations from days, months, years ago.

Reason #10: Your body will reestablish internal stability. All systems will attain normal levels, like the brain, arteries, the breath, bowels, and sleep; they will get easier from each step in the cleansing process.

If you choose to add a helping hand to unstick something, you have an infinite combination of juicing possibilities to select from within this book.

Reason #11: Your body will be awakening from a long sleep. Your entire body will start to process everything effortlessly: neurons and nutrients, together at last. Your aging will slow as you gather yourself to reenter life.

Reason #12: And finally, not that it is the last benefit you will gain from juicing, but simply the final BIG PICTURE benefit for the moment, is this: increased mental clarity.

With so many improvements arriving at once, your brain cannot help but be swept up in the tide of "better, all better."

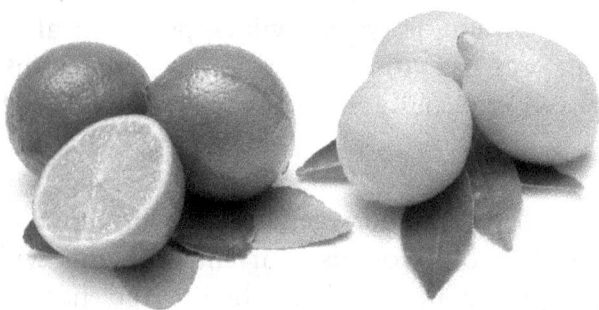

Photo Source: Colourbox.com

PART 1: BENEFITS OF JUICING

Intro

Juicing Is Energy!

Your body needs energy to run and without it you aren't going much of anywhere.

We get energy from the foods we eat. By choosing to juice, you will be utilizing the best source for getting the essential vitamins and minerals your body needs to function.

Ingesting pure foods with no additives or preservatives is where we need to start.

Fresh Fruits And Vegetables

This comes in the form of fresh fruits, tasty vegetables and other healthy plant-based ingredients.

You will soon learn more about the incredible benefits of antioxidants for your system. Fortunately for us, high concentrations of them are found specifically in plants.

While many benefits of juicing have been known for centuries, the process was so labor intensive as to be impractical for the average person on a daily basis.

But finally, and not a moment too soon, science has come to our rescue. A special machine was designed to extract every single ounce of nutrients and energy-satiated components from every item being juiced. With the magic of mass production, such devices are now widely available.

These mechanical works of art will be discussed in full in Chapter 3. Including how to choose your very own. For now we will just call it a juicing machine.

Just to be clear: A juicing machine easily turns pure foods into a pre-digested form, which is perfect for the human body to absorb fully a juice.

Gulping down this powerhouse juice, while the enzymes are at maximum potency is important in yielding a huge nutritional boost to the stomach. Because it is predigested, the stomach can use it immediately 'as is.'

The stomach will happily send the excited nutrients and micro-nutrients to saturate your body cells.

Keep one thing in mind, though, you are not in a race. While juice is at its most potent for about 20 minutes, it's no crime if you want to relax and savor a sip or 2. You will be taking in better nutrition even if you are running a little late, than if you consumed any normal meal.

This, my friends, is where – and when – the healing begins.

The massive influx of beneficial nutrients hits your body, pass unopposed through the digestive system, and rush to every part of your system. The hungry parts get fed, and the damaged parts begin their return journey to health.

But let's not get ahead of ourselves. We have plenty of time to explore the mysteries and marvels of juicing.

Let's launch our adventure with a little orientation.

Why do we want to juice? Here are my top 3 reasons ...

1: Three Big Reasons YOU Should Juice

Reason #1: To Improve Your General Health

It soothes the digestion process by removing the digestive load present with any other type of meal.

Juicing protects you from serious disease by boosting your immune system, giving your body the ability to defend itself.

Once these 2 crucial body systems (digestion and immune) are triggered, the magnified healing process can kick in.

Natural juicing **prevents** disease, stopping it in its tracks.

Juicing will help your body reign supreme by destroying new threats. Serious issues like tumors or cancer can be halted.

Better yet, juicing will help you overcome diseases already present. Things like arthritis, ulcers and clogged arteries will improve. As will heart health.

You are going to need a strong ticker if you want to get out there and run a marathon next year, right?

Invigorating juice also helps lessen the symptoms of other taxing illnesses and conditions.

Bye-Bye Fat Deposits

Losing weight becomes a piece of cake with all those fabulous nutrients flowing through your veins. This further helps you feel great. And it does wonders to your every-day disposition.

The important thing here is that all-natural juicing will give you the joy of weight-loss, without trying. This is fundamental to get the ball rolling for most people. That little win at the start will help you get going.

Let it be known that juicing will also help detoxify your body. In other words, it's like an oil change. It cleans out the system and eliminates the toxic sludge, leaving you feeling even better.

Blood flows with less hindrance and you will immediately notice more energy.

Remember WAY back to when you were a kid? Energy was never an issue. The more you ran around playing, the more you wanted to?

Using energy created more energy. And so it will again, once you are fine-tuned.

Other Juicing Pluses

Juicing on a regular basis will help you release stress and function normally again.

Your arteries will flow clear, so you can say goodbye to heart attacks and strokes any time soon.

Bowels will run full speed ahead. That doesn't sound right, but you know what I mean.

Your breathing and brain will be stronger.

Sleep issues will dissipate. No more counting sheep.

Aesthetically, your skin will smooth out, breakouts will diminish and disappear. Just like you see on those commercials.

Believe it or not, invigorating juicing will help you gain physical endurance and stamina by giving your body the energy it needs to build muscle and burn fat.

Psychological Benefits

Like it or not, you lead with your head.

Juicing is going to keep you feeling pleasant and that will please your therapist.

It will help you feel well overall. It will actually increase your happiness level.

Juicing will also clear your head. This will help you make better decisions in life and that's all good.

Your mood is regulated by the sugar in your blood. You know those nasty ups and downs you experience throughout the day? Just a roller coaster of sugar and caffeine – highs then lows, then repeat until time to drop into bed.

Juicing will stop this. It will level your blood sugars and put you in a constant good mood.

That might be annoying to those around you, but certainly will not be for you.

Those that suffer from sunlight affective disorder (SAD) need not worry about it after juicing.

Whole Body System Benefits

Taking a few moments in your day to juice your nutrients will help tighten and firm your skin, which is the largest organ in your body. The aging process will be slowed.

Not the fountain of youth, but a nice start.

Juicing will also help improve muscle tone and improve your ability to stretch, which reduces troublesome aches and pains. It helps 'lubricate' your system, for lack of a better word. Helping your body operate with less squeaks.

You can forget about your cholesterol level, because juicing is a positive there, too, reducing it to a safe range.

We're not going to stop here. There is much more to be said in favor of juicing.

Reason #2: To Maintain Your Well-Being

Fact is that very few people in the world today consume enough fruits and vegetables.

But with juicing, it is almost effortless. You toss your fresh fruits into a juicing machine and start it up.

In a few minutes you have a tasty drink, teeming with enzymes, nutrients, vitamins and minerals.

Bring it on.

Physical Health Benefits Of Juicing

Ah, where to start.

Juicing will help improve digestion. We've touched on this before. Think about it for a minute. You don't need to chew or breakdown food, and your stomach doesn't need to either.

The work has already been done ... by your juicing machine. All you have to do is DRINK UP.

With Juicing You Get:

- Fast results – nutrients are available to be soaked up by your body's systems.
- More energy – getting important vitamins and minerals increases energy.
- More nutrients are assimilated – nutrients don't flush through your system, they stick.
- Time saved – 5 minutes for preparation.
- Healthier hair – nutrients go to all body parts, including hair and nails.

- Stronger bones – studies show that juicing strengthens bones.

- A cleaner liver – your liver cleans your system. If it slows down, toxins build in your body.

- Weight-loss – probably the most popular benefit because it's painless.

- A better immune system. The huge doses of antioxidants quickly strengthen your immune system.

- Slower aging process – throw out those expensive creams; juice some blackberries and blueberries instead. They are a great source of vitamins C, E and other antioxidants to help prevent skin aging and those dreaded wrinkles.

- Better heart health – Vitamin C and E help prevent blood from sticking and clotting in the arteries and they lower triglycerides. Potassium and magnesium are critical for great heart function and avoiding arrhythmia.

- Cancer prevention – a famous benefit of juicing, for sure. Some say that juicing can even reverse cancer.

- Better brain function – thinking straighter can't hurt.

- Improved joint function – especially important as we age.

- Reduced arthritis pain – another common disease that juicing can take a bite out of.

- Reduced inflammation – juicing helps with the pain associated with inflammation.

- More blood cells – we can always use more of these and juicing gives you just that.

This is all made possible, in part, by chlorophyll, the secret weapon from plants.

Sidebar:

Before we continue. I need to explain a new feature that is coming to you very soon – the Glossary reference. To make the main section of the book easy to read, I've moved the more scientifically dense information into the Glossary at the back of the book. It is well worth your time to pause and take a 'once-over' look when you see the Glossary indicator.

If you see a word with a superscript (like this: "Chlorophyll[5]"), that means there is a complete discussion in the Glossary at the end of the book. I recommend that you check out the Glossary for at least the first few references. Then decide if you want those extra details.

I just wanted to let you know, because your opportunity is coming real **soon**.

·❖·◆·❖·

Juice Contains:

1. Chlorophyll[5] – a great nutrient that is typically found in plants that yield a characteristic green juice. [Did you check out that Glossary reference? Oops, here comes another.]

2. Antioxidants[3] – A wide array of components necessary for healthy functioning of cells and various tissues of the body. You really can't live without these compounds.

3. Proteins[12] – Fruit and vegetable juices are usually considered a poor source of protein. But don't let that get you down, because they contain a nice variety of amino acids for your body to process, in order to create ... protein. Amino Acids[1] are the building blocks of proteins in the body and we need them to create structurally correct proteins.

4. Carbohydrates[4] – They come in 3 main forms:

- Simple sugars.
- Complex carbohydrates.
- Fiber.

Fruits tend to have more simple sugars than vegetables do. Think sweeter.

Most fruits and vegetables provide carbohydrates, but you'll find an abundance of them in starchy vegetables like potatoes, corn, and rice.

Fresh juice contains proteins, carbohydrates, essential fatty acids, vitamins, & minerals in a form your body can easily take up.

5. Essential Fatty Acids[7] – In general, fruits are relatively low in fats. But there are some fatty acids found in fruits which are absolutely essential to life. They are called 'essential' because they can't be made by your body – you have to get them from your diet.

6. Vitamins[13] – Juices are excellent sources of soluble vitamins, including A, C, D, E, K and B-Complex.

7. Minerals[10] – Plants extract minerals from the soil through their roots. Then they combine those with organic compounds within their tissues. The resulting mineral products are easily taken in by your body. Hence, plants are an excellent source of minerals.

You'll find plenty of goodies like: chloride, sodium, sulfur, potassium, aluminum, chromium, copper, cobalt, fluoride, iron, and zinc. Enough to build a healthy body ... or a Lear jet.

8. Enzymes[6] – In order for food to be digested by your body, enzymes are required. This relationship is a 'live' one and the

best foods for this process are ones that already come with their own enzymes, like vegetable juices.

Fresh fruit and vegetable juices are excellent sources of enzymes.

9. Phytochemicals[11] – Phytochemicals are pigments and compounds found in plants that together create the plant's signature smell, color and flavor.

Plants have thousands of different kinds of phytochemicals, but only a handful has been studied to date.

Psychological Benefits Of Juicing

Juicing is going to help you:

- Feel fantastic.
- Be less moody.
- Avoid depression.

Improve your sense of well-being.

A nice fresh glass of juice is all it takes to tell your brain that everything is fine.

To Sum Up

There are many mental and physical advantages that come from juicing.

You'll lose weight and gain confidence.

Your body will boast endless stores of positive energy.

Weight will melt, leaving you feeling spectacular and looking amazing.

You will replenish lost stores of nutrients your body needs to fight off the 'free-radicals' of the world.

And that's just to start.

Let's see what's in store when it comes to diseases.

Reason #3: To Prevent Disease

Juices are loaded with nutrients, essential vitamins and minerals that start the healing process within minutes. Having a diet high in fruits and veggies will help prevent a wide range of ailments. Some of which are deadly.

Because these natural juices are easily processed and digested, they are awesome for preventing digestive issues.

Type 2 diabetics who drink fresh juice daily can *sometimes* dramatically decrease their insulin consumption. Just watch the sugar content.

What are the specific benefits of juicing for disease prevention?

Benefits

Popping the fruits and veggies into the juicer will help you disease-wise by:

- Eliminating toxic chemicals.
- Getting rid of waste products.
- Reducing cholesterol.
- Lowering high blood pressure.
- Getting your daily requirements of fruits and vegetables.
- Dissolving kidney stones.
- Detoxifying the liver, gallbladder, kidneys, heart and brain.
- Boosting your immune system function.
- Preventing colds, flu and other infectious diseases.
- Reversing blocked arteries.
- Preventing heart attacks.
- Halting tumor growth.

- Destroying cancer cells.

Regular juicing can enhance overall health.

Add to this, phytochemicals may well hold the keys to preventing:

- Cancer.
- Heart Disease.
- Asthma.
- Arthritis.
- Allergies.

Amazing … or preposterous? You be the judge.

First, let's look at cancer prevention:

Broccoli contains a substance that helps prevent and may even cure breast cancer. Likewise, citrus fruits have substances that assist in the removal of carcinogens, which decreases the chance of getting cancer.

Looking at grapes, they contain a chemical that helps protect the cell from DNA damage. And several green veggies have substances that offer cancer protection too.

The mind-blower is that a simple tomato has over 10,000 chemical compounds in it. **One** of which is the awesome 'phytochemicals,' mentioned before.

The question is, what will the other 9,999 compounds do for you?

It really is hard to put into words just how extremely beneficial juicing fresh fruits and vegetables is, mentally, physically and emotionally. But don't think that's going to stop me from trying.

Your mind is extremely powerful.

If you 'think' you are going to be too tired, you will be. If you believe you are going to lose the tennis game, you likely will.

Juicing will get your body into a pleasant state. This is going to make you happy and better able to deal with work and relationships in a positive light, instead of instinctively pulling out the boxing gloves.

Just knowing the glass is half-full is going to make your life something you bounce out of bed in the morning for, rather than hit the snooze button.

Who knows, you may even start enjoying your day!

OK class ... now we're going to move on to the basics of juicing. Sound good?

Oran Kangas

2: Learn The Basics Of Juicing

Intro

We are going to talk about the most basic thing in juicing: why.

Without understand why, and having your own personal why, you will quit. Not just juicing, but any new program. When things are shiny and new, it is easy to jump aboard and try things.

Just look at all the discarded stuff you have lying about your abode. It all sounded so good. It looked so good. You jumped in. And jumped right back out. Right?

Juicing is NOT going to be like that. Not if I can help it.

I want you to fully understand what you are getting into and why you would and should want to.

We are going to examine this from various perspectives:

1. Why juicing works.
2. Your primary goal in juicing.
3. The procedural steps of juicing.
4. Juicing ingredients you will use.
5. Alkalizing foods.

Why And How Juicing Works

WHY ME? Why on Earth would I actually want to consider juicing?

Back To Bio 101

Plants put their roots in the ground, extract minerals and store them in their cell walls. They convert dirt to bio-available minerals, trace minerals and other nutrients.

Fresh vegetables and fruits are not just any old weeds, though.

They are especially rich in plan enzymes, phytonutrients, antioxidants, and vitamins. This is in addition to the normal complement of minerals and other goodies they have stored in their little green bellies.

The nutritional values of these plants you ingest are extremely **beneficial** to your body. This raw produce is filled with important, plant derived enzymes.

Why is this important? I'm glad you asked, because enzymes: initiate, direct, or accelerate almost every chemical reaction in life.

Powerful is an understatement.

They are, however, also very fragile the cooking process kills them.

So are we stuck with eating dead chickens or chewing on grass? NO.

I welcome you to the new age.

While our bodies are efficient at processing food, our digestive system can't extract nutrients until it is ground up. Even then, an enormous amount of energy goes into the nutrient rendering process. That's the price we pay for being omnivores (able to eat anything).

And now, making its GRAND entrance from your cluttered corner kitchen cupboard is the 'Magic' juicing machine. (applause)

Science has invented the perfect way to turn those nutrient filled organic plants (yummy), into something the human body can easily process, juice.

This machine chews the plants up for us, just like a bird does for her young, literally pulverizing the entire plant and its tough cell walls.

The Result

Unleashed nutrients we would otherwise never experience.

Juicing gives you the high concentration of vital vitamins and micro-nutrients previously held prisoner in the plant cell walls. It releases nutrients we wouldn't normally digest, like the skin and seeds which are now, usually, available to us.

For Bonus Points

The enzymes are still alive and working hard as you drink away.

Juicing is simply the easiest way to get all your recommended daily servings of fruits and vegetables. That's 5 fruits and 3 vegetables, right?

Most people don't get anywhere near those numbers. But it is easy, even tasty with fresh juices.

Juicing yields the highest density of nutrients per calorie. Very impressive.

Juicing gives your body the nutrients it craves and a mountain of wealth is absorbed directly into your bloodstream. Your anxiously awaiting internal organs are going to be very, very happy.

You can make all sorts of different tasty juices by combining what you like and what you aren't so fond of. How so? There are amazing fruits and vegetables that will mask just about any flavor.

Have fun! Experiment and create your personalized juices.

Why Not Just Buy Pre-Made Fresh Juices?

Because they are dead!

The enzymes so incredibly important for your body have a life span of only a few hours after they are processed.

Use it or lose it could never ring truer.

Benefits Of Juicing:

- Prevents or cures numerous diseases and illnesses.
- Invigorates immediately.
- Improves digestive system.
- Calms.
- Makes reaching the centurion club (age 100) possible.
- Saves time, so being busy is no longer an excuse.
- Soothes your stomach.
- Gives more nutrients than eating the fruit or vegetable whole.
- Prevents crashes after chugging (think alcohol, coffee).
- Smooths skin and diminishes wrinkles.
- Promotes healing.
- Detoxifies your body naturally.

We are going to talk briefly about ...

Detoxification

That is the elimination of accumulated toxic waste stores from your body. Raw juices are the best way to detoxify your body, often reversing the deadly degenerative effects of a poor diet. Many have a laxative effect that encourages additional detoxification of your body.

Good news for you.

Raw juices usually take only 10-20 minutes to pass through an empty stomach. Ideally, you should drink on an empty stomach when juicing. Since there is no other food for the juice to compete with, your gut can more easily recognize that the nutrients are already broken down and quickly pass them through for absorption.

Hydration

Did you know that by the time you figure out you are thirsty, you are already dehydrated? (When that yucky, pasty taste hits, you are long past due.)

Fruits and veggies provide 1 more crucial item to your health – WATER.

65% of human body cells are comprised of water. Your noggin is 80% water. (I know some people who are approaching 100%, if ya know what I mean.)

It goes without saying that most folks don't get enough water. But I said it, anyway.

Even if we drink soda, tea, coffee or alcoholic drinks, most of that gets eliminated before our bodies can use it.

The Solution?

Vegetable and fruit juices, filled with fresh, unpolluted water.

Components

Juices are filled with antioxidants.

They have a great supply of vital minerals such as: iron, copper, potassium, sodium, iodine and magnesium.

Examples:
- Citrus fruits provide Vitamin C.
- Carrot juice contains Vitamin A & beta-carotene.
- Green juices provide a great supply of Vitamin E.
- Celery juice treats allergies.
- Spinach and kale often are used to treat anemia.
- Dandelion greens and pineapple juices are great for rheumatoid arthritis.

I'll bet all this philosophical insight about juicing has flicked your excitement switch. Well, just wait until you see what is next!

Get A Goal

Life is all about goals and focus. A goal is something to work towards, an external motivator to help you make positive internal changes.

Goals In Juicing?

Sound a little bit weird? Just think of it as a plan. By now you've already learned that juicing is incredibly positive for your mind and body.

It's important that you figure out what your particular goals are in juicing. This way you can start making them happen. Until the 'happening' happens, goals are a meaningless generality.

Are your planning a juicing detox? Do you want to start adding juicing into your life 2 times a day? Do you want to make juicing your daily focus? Would you like to drop 20 pounds?

Such questions need to be asked and answered, if you are going to set 'successful' goals.

Baby Steps First

Maybe you want to:

- Lose weight.
- Relieve a health issue.
- Improve your thinking.
- Alleviate body pain.
- Improve your energy.
- Prevent illness.
- Battle the aging process.
- OR all of the above.

There are many excellent reasons for adopting juicing into your lifestyle. Figure yours out and we can proceed to actually creating some actionable juicing goals.

How Are You Going To Reach Your Goals?

A commitment is needed.

This may sound like a given, but saying and doing are 2 different things. Until you commit to an action AND a schedule, your results will be sporadic, at best.

Commit to juicing and mean it. If you are not deadly serious in your commitment, the ultimate consequences to your body just might be **seriously deadly.** Think about it.

You need to make a list. No need to check it twice.

You are probably going to need a juice machine (we'll get to that soon). Just jot it down. Recipes (coming up real soon now), and lots of fresh fruits. That's what you will need to play this game. Are you a player?

Well, maybe 1 more thing: a bathroom nearby. Actually the bathroom may not be a serious factor at all. Juicing affects people differently. Some get diarrhea, others get constipated. Many notice no change at all in that department. Wherever you land on that factor, it's no big deal. It will pass, so to speak.

With a list of your goal(s) and your 'necessary equipment,' you have a 'visual' to help get your healthy new juicing habit into motion. If you need to, stick it on your bathroom mirror as a reminder.

Do It

Be fair to yourself.

Sure, you are excited and want to drop a few pounds in the first week. Fair enough.

But you need to set yourself up for success. Make sure you can reach your goals. Otherwise, you are setting yourself up to fail.

Create a support system. This is very important for success. Tell people about your new juicing lifestyle. It's easy to give up on yourself. But when you have someone else to answer to, it's a different story.

Stupid as that is. Why are we okay with letting ourselves down? That's just wrong, don't you think?

Onward.

It's OK to fall off the horse. Get back on.

I don't care who you are. If you are going to succeed you have to keep trying.

Expect hiccups on the road to juicing wellness. They are inevitable.

If you happen to go away for the weekend and forget your juicer. **Don't Quit.**

When you get back, just forget about the interruption. There's no use crying over spilt milk.

Get your juicer out and get to it with more determination than ever.

Understand this isn't about punishment and reward.

Every single time you juice, you are giving your body the enzymes it needs to be at its best. Healthy and strong, and fighting to stay that way.

That is how you need to look at it.

So if you only remember 1 thing about goals, make it this:

Start juicing. Keep juicing. Make juicing a habit.

OK, that was 3 things.

Recap

- Decide EXACTLY what you want to accomplish.
- Make sure you have a DETAILED plan in place.
- Have support people to hold you accountable.
- EXPECT setbacks.
- Practice, practice, practice.

Pretty simple, right? Now let's move on to doing. It's time to learn HOW to juice and soon after you are going to start reaping the rewards.

Procedure – How To Do It

There are a multitude of ways to juice fruits and vegetables.

Regardless which extraction method is used, your organic produce needs some prepping before juicing.

Ingredient Preparation:

Purchase organic produce if at all possible. If you have a local farmers market that is ideal.

Organic fruits and vegetables are a priority for juicing! After all, who wants pesticides, herbicides, synthetic fertilizers, and who knows what else in their life giving juice?

To get organic produce, the most cost effective way is usually to shop at a local farmers market. If that is not an option, then I suggest you adjust your thinking and your budget to make health your #1 priority. Most grocery stores now carry organic versions of produce, they just charge too much for it.

But too much relative to what? Sickness, disease, illness are all very expensive conditions. If you factor in the value of avoiding the lost wages and cost of medicine, to say nothing of the misery involved, you may find it really pays to go organic.

Due to the wide-spread practice of toxic spraying, there are some products that you really, really should consume only in organic form. In the fruit department, we have:

apples, cherries, grapes, nectarines, papaya, peaches, pears, and strawberries. Over in the veggies aisle: bell peppers, carrots, celery, corn, kale, lettuce, and spinach.

These products are especially likely to have been toxically treated. You really don't want that chemical residue going through your juicer and your body.

SHOCKER: It's takes A LOT of fruits and veggies to get a glass of fresh juice. That is why they are so loaded with vitamins, minerals, and other nutrients. Which gives you energy like you wouldn't believe.

Water Filters

A similar case can be made regarding water. Water from the tap generally contains all sorts of impurities. And then the treatment plants let loose their barrage of chemicals to kill those impurities.

Well, impurities may not be the only casualty of that war. It's better to be safely filtered, than sorry you are drinking that sludge.

You need to start thinking about water filters. Filters come in a vast array of choices, capabilities and price ranges. The best rule of thumb is to buy the best you can afford. You will not only be safer, but you will notice a huge leap in taste satisfaction.

Preparation

Preparation of your soon to be a juice ingredients should occur immediately before you are ready to drink it, to insure maximum nutrition.

Rinse your produce off before using. Dirt has an awful aftertaste.

Use a vegetable brush to remove dirt, debris, and any chemical residues from the surface of ingredients.

Cut off any bruised or spoiled spots, as they can affect taste and clarity. Rotten tastes rotten.

Only peel if you have to. Don't forget that there are many vitamins and minerals in the skin.

In general, the seeds are good, except remove the stones from fruit, seeds from papaya, and pips from apples.

Of course, you will need to slice your fresh produce so it fits into your juicer, and away you go. For some machines, that will be no slicing at all.

Juicing

Fill your juicer up and press start.

Good juicers will mulch everything up, pulverizing ingredients, thereby extracting nearly every drop of juice to give you the benefit of all the nutrients.

Now enjoy. The oxidation process happens fast and you don't want to lose those benefits you just created. Drink within 20 minutes for the best effects.

Time for cleanup. The fun part. Do it right away and save some extra scrubbing. (Check out the Maintenance Chapter for more enlightenment.) If you procrastinate, you will pay a price in juicing as in life.

Now we are getting to the good stuff. Time to figure out **what** you should be juicing.

Elements – Which Juices Play Nice Together

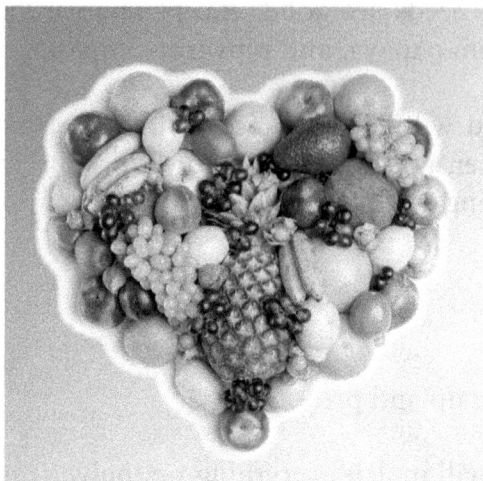

Photo Source: colourbox.com

First lesson – there are juicy fruits and there are not-so-juicy fruits. Avocados, bananas, and strawberries don't have a lot of juice in them, so when juicing, it works best to combine them with 'juicier' fruits and juices.

Apples, cantaloupe, grapefruit, grapes, oranges, peaches, pears and watermelon are 'Gold Medal' juicers. YUM!

Lesson 2 – pay attention to texture. Like a thicker drink? Go for soft fruits, like peaches and pears. Prefer a thinner, smoother beverage? Pulverize some harder fruits, like apples.

Combine Fruits And Vegetables

It works best to juice fruits and veggies apart to start because different stomach acids and enzymes are used to digest fruits and vegetables. Your body will not ingest as many nutrients as a result. Plus, you could get an upset tummy.

NOTE: This is a prevalent THEORY. Your results may be different. Mine were. I juice with abandon, my stomach sorts things out, and we're all just fine. The cardinal rule is pay attention to your body, not someone else's theory. Then you can make your own rules.

There is one product that everyone can agree on ...

The Apple

An apple is an exception to the above theory. Apples are neutral in the produce wars. You can use them with other fruits or with vegetables to make the juice taste sweeter. They are a fruit which lives in blissful harmony with all fruits and vegetables. No worries with mixing there.

We could all take a lesson from the apple.

Great Juicing Bases

- Apples and carrots.
- Apples, oranges and carrots.
- Carrots, apples and beetroot or pineapple.
- Spinach, carrots and apples or pears.
- Lemons, limes and oranges.

These are all terrific combinations to start with. The keys are to be **creative** and **experiment**. Time to live on the edge. Show your true colors!

But start simple. Don't go getting complicated on me. One recipe to start with. Be patient.

After you have that recipe fine-tuned, you're free to spice things up a notch or 2.

Start slow and SIP your fresh juice. Have a glass to start each meal, so that your body can get used to all the goodness you're providing. Honest.

It won't take long before you can juice here, there and everywhere!

Now I know that the veggies are good for your body. But let's face it. Fruits taste a whole lot better. My 'professional' advice to you is steer more to the fruits first. Then SLOWLY implement some veggies.

Before you know it, you'll be able to switch hit successfully whenever you choose.

Trust me. You'll find your balance.

Summation:

Experiment to find what your body tolerates best. Probably all fruit juices can be combined. Apple works great with just about any juicing drink.

It is when you come to mixing veggies and fruits that things can get more complicated. Some will simply say you shouldn't. I say you shouldn't take their word for it. Trust your own body.

Alkalizing Foods – For Better Body Balance

Another important concept is alkalizing foods, which are usually lacking in normal diets. Luckily this is reversible by simply changing the PH in your body from acidic to alkaline-based. This is easily done through normal juicing, juice fasting, and eating healthier foods.

Make your juicer sweat, while you sit back and enjoy.

Did you know plant juice is the optimum source of nutrition for humans? No other source of nutrition delivers valuable nutrients as quickly as the natural juice of fruits and vegetables.

It provides them in their living, organic, alkaline, whole, complete and balanced form(s).

Science tells us that the ideal balance for the human body is 80% alkaline and 20% acid. Our bodies have better health and vitality when at or near these levels. This points us toward the crop of broccoli for some of our juicing, not just the apple orchard!

A long time ago, everyone ate fresh vegetables daily, making it easy to maintain such percentages. However, today alkaline containing nutrition is much harder to come by for most people. Think fast food joints, vending machines, box dinners, all of which do not do your body good!

Our bodies are mostly water and our PH levels need to be internally neutral in order to function properly. When we accumulate too much acid in our system, more than our body can get rid of, we become overly acidic, leading to:

- Gout.
- Obesity.
- Stomach disorders.

- Digestion problems.

- Irritable bowel syndrome.

- Immune deficiencies.

- Cell death.

- Bodily systems slowing.

- Decay setting in from the inside out.

- Yeasts and fungi start growing, feeding on sugar and acid, which deteriorates the body further.

- Sickness that turns serious quickly.

- Chronic aches and pains.

- Low energy.

- Poor sleep.

- Trouble focusing and remembering.

- Increased chance of developing arthritis.

- Longer illnesses, due to our poor immune systems.

Beneficial Effects

Neutralizing the acid in our body through juicing the correct healthy foods will help build energy stores, strengthen our body internally and help it to better fight off serious disease and illness.

Examples

Greens, veggies, non-sweet fruits, specific grains and nuts, and other whole and natural foods are prime examples of excellent alkalizing foods.

OK. You've done all the prep work. Now we're going to get you started.

Let's look at HOW to do juicing.

PART 2: HOW TO GET STARTED

Intro

What shall we talk about next?

How about getting started the right way? Sound good?

First Is Equipment:
- Types to choose from.
- How to select a juicer.
- Maintaining a juicer.
- Getting some accessories.

Then It's On To Types Of INGREDIENTS:
- Fruits.
- Berries.
- Melons.
- Spices.
- Sweeteners.

Then We'll Close Off With Avoiding Juice Boredom:
- Substitutions.
- Smoothies.
- Recycling pulp with frozen treats.
- Naming.

3: Equip Yourself

Intro

We are going to look into juicing equipment now. The types available, proper maintenance, what accessories you will want (now and later), and end with a selection guide to picking out your own juicer.

Exciting stuff ahead: You're going to see all the types of equipment available for you to buy.

There are many brands within the general types of juicing machines you can purchase. The one you choose will affect your long-term success, so,

PAY ATTENTION! ... please?

Juicing Equipment TYPES Available

It goes without saying, yet I shall say it, you need to invest in a *good* juicer. Think of it as a long term healthy life insurance policy.

One thing for certain is:

After having freshly juiced juice you will NEVER willingly go back the store-bought stuff. That is usually pasteurized, which destroys many of the nutrients. Also, the quality of the produce that goes into store bought juice is much lower than our standards.

The Name Game

The juicing equipment marketplace can be summed up in 1 word: Confusing. There are sooo many different juicers vying for consideration and each tries to out-claim the other.

Further muddling the situation is the constant name swapping, for no good reason.

Let me simplify for you:

- Juicer = Juice Machine = Juice Extractor = Juice Fountain.
- Masticating (sounds dangerous) = Single Gear.
- Triturating = Twin Gear.

With that out of the way, here are 3 fun ways to group juicers:

- The good, the bad and the ... special.

To be thorough, I'll talk about all of them below, but I'm guessing you want to hear about the good ones first.

The Good

Good juicers fall into 3 categories:

1. Centrifugal.
2. Masticating.
3. Triturating.

Don't be intimidated, those terms just describe their methods of separating juice from pulp.

I'll describe first and sum up at the end ... fair enough?

Centrifugal Juicer

A centrifugal juicer shreds ingredients with sharp blades, and then spins out the juice at a high speed, which then drips down to a collection pool. The bits of skin, seeds and other pulp are separated and usually tossed out the juicer's back door, into an awaiting container.

The juice yield is less from this form of extraction, with pulp remaining moist with juice waste.

Due to increased oxidation inherent in the process, the juice should be consumed sooner.

The majority of juicers are of this type. You can find them everywhere. And they generally do an okay job juicing greens, however wheat grass is beyond them.

Pluses
- They are fast.
- Usually the cheapest.
- Great for newbies.
- Easy to clean.

- Easy to use.

Negatives
- Noisy.
- They get very hot, which kills off some of the enzymes and antioxidants.
- NOT at their best when juicing herbs or leafy greens.
- Don't even bother trying wheat grass.

Masticating Juicer

Want healthier – use this. If your gut is telling you that serious juicing is in your future, a masticating juicer is likely right for you.

Chewing ... grinding ... crushing: that's what this juicer is all about. Then it pushes the product through a wire mesh with attitude.

Pluses
- If you had to use one word, it's sturdy.
- They are excellent for pulverizing most fruits, hard vegetables, grains, leafy greens, and ... even WHEAT GRASS.
- Less heat than the centrifugal, so a better juice quality is the result.
- It can turn nuts into creamy nut butter.
- It is great for making baby foods and sorbets.

Of course there's always a 'but.'

Negatives
- Costs more.
- Takes up more space (but not a lot more).

- Takes longer to juice.

Some models require more prep and cleaning, and might get clogged more often. So don't buy those models.

The Triturating Juicer

It uses a 2 step process: Crushing first. Pressing second. The veggies pass through the twin gears and are squeezed, chewed, ground up, and spat out (figuratively speaking).

These juicers are the gold standard of the 3 main types.

Pluses

- You get even more fiber, enzymes, vitamins, and trace minerals than from a masticating juicer.
- It intentionally works at a very slow speed, which makes it slightly more effective at producing juice.
- It has a magnetic and bio-ceramic technology that slows oxidation, which helps if you store juice.
- It's the quietest of all.
- You can make: sauces, baby foods, nut butters, fruit ice creams, and fruit sorbets.
- Wheat grass is a cinch.

Negatives

- They are the slowest.
- They are expensive.
- And a little harder to clean.

That finishes the Good category. Now for the dark side of juicing.

The Bad

It's time for a few laughs. The award for the worst engineering idea goes to ...

The Steam Juicer (applause please)

Steam juicers essentially cook your fruits and vegetables ... to death. After which they proceed to collect the dead juices that dribble through the machine.

You get ...

Decaying vegetative matter in a liquid form. Can I get a collective YUCK?

Let's see a show of hands for how many people want one of those.

Nobody? Then let's look at the infamous ...

Food Processor

Some models have a juicing attachment to remove fiber from juicing ingredients during the squishing process.

Verdict? Guilty ... of being designed for an entirely different purpose.

You might use this if you **seldom** make fresh juices and already own one. But to buy it specifically to juice would be really dumb.

The Special

Hydraulic Juicer Press

If you can afford it and can find one, GO FOR IT.

Designed for commercial use, it presses produce like no other, to squeeze out every ounce of juice. Giving you all the nutrients and leaving nothing behind.

It has been dubbed the most effective juicer known to man.

It's about 10 steps above the rest, but you'd be hard 'pressed' to find it in any store. (Sorry, couldn't resist.)

Blender

So what about a normal blender?

The main difference between a blender and a juicer is that a blender has no way to separate the fiber and the juice. It doesn't even try. You just don't get 'pulp-free' with a blender.

The separation process is beneficial because it lets your body digest juice without utilizing much energy, which is precisely *because* there is little fiber to break down.

Although blenders don't make great juices, they do have a knack for great smoothies.

Juicers give you only the nutrients – blenders give you fiber. If you are *primarily* looking for the benefits of pulp (and there definitely are many, which I will discuss later), then a blender is a good option.

Another plus for the blender is that, on average, they are quicker and easier to clean.

Actually, I recommend and use both. I fit the equipment to my needs, as everyone should. For juice, it's a juicer; for smoothies, it's a blender.

Since I seldom crave a smoothie, I count myself in the juicer camp, but that in no way makes me anti-blender.

Citrus Juicer

This item hones in on 1 thing, juicing citrus.

Perhaps after you become a juicing veteran, you will one day see the point of a dedicated citrus juicer. So far, I don't.

Manual Juicers

Electricity ... where are you? This is so 19th century.

To Recap

There are 3 main types of juicers to consider buying:

Centrifugal – loudest, fastest, cheapest, least nutrients, easy clean.

Masticating – bigger, slower, more expensive, more nutrients.

Triturating – biggest, slowest, most money, most nutrients.

Which sounds best to you? OK, you don't have to decide just yet. You have 1 more section before picking up that phone.

How To Pick YOUR Juicer

In juicer selection, the following factors should be considered:

Ease Of Use

Easy: means you're going to **use** it. Hard: you're going to **store** it.

The best juicer is the one that you will actually use. Ease of use is far more important than you think it will be. Trust me on this.

Juicing Speed

We are an impatient breed. Centrifugal juicers are the fastest. But that creates more problems than it solves:

- Noise – annoys the cat.
- Heat – destroys the enzymes you are looking for.
- Air – increases oxidation.

If you can't stand the heat, get out of the kitchen, or choose another juicer.

Speed really is bad for you.

Types Of Produce

- Some juicers work better with 'problem' ingredients:
- Leafy greens, soft fruits, many vegetables, and the ever troublesome wheat grass.
- Vegetables have fibrous, 'tough' cell walls, which require more gusto in the extraction method.

The masticating and triturating juicers were designed especially for handling the above troublemakers. Of course, they are going to make you dig a little deeper in your pocket.

The Opening Size

Some juicers have a wide feeding chute.

That is handy because it reduces prep (chopping) time.

Quality Of Juice

Centrifugal = poorer quality juice.

Masticating = better quality juice.

Triturating = best quality juice.

Oxidation

Centrifugal heats up and causes oxidation ... not good. But not too bad, if you drink fairly quickly.

Triturating juicers are slower, which isn't good for enzyme levels either. BUT they don't heat up. So those 2 factors balance out.

30 minutes is considered the enzyme half-life, meaning half are lost every half hour. So storage should be a last resort.

Yield

Better juicers give you more juice.

Noise Level

Centrifugal, think truck. Masticating and trituration, more like an electric can opener.

Versatility

You can do a whole lot more with a masticating juicer. End of story.

Replacement Parts

This can be a pain in the rear pocket. Research before ordering to make sure you can get future parts without being gouged.

Durability And Reliability

You get what you pay for. Usually. On-line reviews are a great way to check this out.

Power

Like a truck, the more powerful the motor, the less it has to work to get the job done, and the longer it will generally last.

BUT power is measured in watts, not RPM. A motor rating of 450 watts or greater is recommended. The thing you need to be concerned about when purchasing a cheap machine is motor power. Weak motors won't cut it, or juice it ... for long.

Price

Of course, price is important, but the most expensive isn't necessarily the best ... for you. If you are just testing out the juicing idea, don't buy the best juicer out there. Not yet; in other words, be sure before you invest a lot.

Warranty/Guarantee

3 years MINIMUM. Some juicers go up to 15 years. Wow. Better warranty = greater faith by the manufacturer.

Pulp: Ejection Or Not

Juicers come in 2 types: pulp-ejection and non-pulp ejection.

Pretty self-explanatory, ejection machines send the pulp into a separate container during juicing. That is good if you juice in large quantities. With non-ejectors, you need to stop after 1 quart to clean it out.

Paper filters make cleaning a lot easier and you are rewarded with a finely strained juice.

I'm all for saving work. I went for an ejection model. But it's a close call, either way.

Portability

If you travel a lot, smaller is handy. Keep in mind, this generally means less power.

Summation

That is a heap of facts to process. Let's simplify way down:

- If you aren't sure about juicing and money is an issue, go centrifugal.
- If business was good this year, go triturating.
- For everyone else, go masticating.

Final Selection Process

1. Select your type: centrifugal, masticating, or triturating. You should know this by now.

2. Prioritize the above criteria according to your needs.

3. Then go online to get some reviews. (I like to use Amazon because they stock darned near everything and they have a bazillion customers. So lots of unbiased product reviews.)

4. Compare the highest rated models to your prioritized criteria

5. That should help you quickly hone in on the right manufacturer/model for your needs.

Now it's deal time. Who will ship that bright shiny machine at the best price? Again, I used my trusty computer to search the internet.

Just type in that model number from above and out jumps a whole batch of virtual salesmen. Select a vendor with a great price and good reviews regarding delivery.

Keep in mind that you are after the juicer that best suits *your* juicing purpose.

That's really all there is to it. You could agonize over this decision for days, and still not be any better prepared than you are right NOW.

So, it's time to pick one. Pull out a quarter and flip it, if that's what it takes.

Now ... pick up the phone. It's okay if your hand is shaking. Dial. That's good. And ... place that juicer order. The good life is calling.

Maintenance – Treat It Right And It Will Treat You Right

While we're waiting for it to arrive, let's continue learning. Then when your juicing machine arrives at your front doorstep, you'll be ready to juice.

Juicers are awesome machines. But if you neglect to clean them properly, they will become useful in your child's science class when they are studying fungi and molds.

Solution: Simply clean it immediately after use and forget it.

I will not lie. Cleaning is a pain, but it's not so bad if you do it right away.

Actually, it takes me 3 minutes to disassemble, clean, and reassemble my juicer (I timed it).

If you need to, leave it in the sink to soak, and clean it later. It's not a big deal, unless you avoid it.

Be Clean And Safe

Of course your counter tops, cutting boards and any utensils that come in contact with your fresh produce need to be cleaned thoroughly. And NOT the cheating way, by just rising in warm water cither (I know you do it).

It's best to rinse and sanitize them in a mild bleach solution and then air dry them.

Note: A good eco-friendly choice is "oxygen bleach." It safely disinfects, removes stains, and comes in liquid or powder form. Regular bleach uses the highly toxic sodium hypochlorite as the cleansing agent.

Now we're going to scoot through the cleaning steps ... so bare (sic) with me.

Cleaning Supplies:

- Plastic spoon.
- Towel.
- Scouring sponge.
- Nylon cleaning brushes.
- Small pipe cleaning brush.
- Liquid dish washing detergent.
- Oxygen bleach.

As soon as you've finished juicing, turn the juicer off and unplug the cord (safety first).

Take your juicer apart – it's easy, or you bought the wrong machine. If there is a pulp container, remove it and empty the contents into the compost or trash (if you must).

Use the plastic spoon to scrap away any excess pulp. Tip: It helps to place a freezer bag into the pulp collector for easy cleaning purposes.

Carefully remove the motor base and set it aside. Wipe it with a dirty sponge ... kidding. Use a CLEAN damp one, please. Do NOT put the motor in water, unless you want to go buy a new juicer just for fun.

Watch your fingers if there are blades involved, cuz you don't want to lose one!

Fill the sink with soapy hot water and a few drops of oxy-bleach, and let the parts soak. If there are blocked holes in the filter basket, just soak the basket in hot water with a few capfuls of lemon juice. Lemon juice also works for stains.

For tough to reach spots, use a pipe cleaning brush.

Rinse each part under hot water after soaking and air dry on a towel. When dry, reassemble and store in your juicer storage area. See, easy.

Blade Notes (If your juicer has blades, like the Centrifugal models): Remove blade and use a soft brush to clean it gently. Be careful, very sharp. Inspect regularly and make sure it is in great working order, because it is the key to your juicing.

Juicer Servicing

From time-to-time, all good equipment needs a once over at the shop.

Your best bet is to have a look at the owner's manual, which of course you've read thoroughly. Here it should tell you how often it needs a 'real' servicing.

Important Info To Record In A Safe Place:

- Where are you putting the owner's manual?
- When does the 'guarantee' expire? Murphy's Law says your machine is going to fly apart the day AFTER. Avoid this with a thorough testing a month before d-day and you should be good to go.
- When does the manual say to have it serviced?
- Can you have it serviced locally? If so, you can save time and shipping costs.
- Write down the email address and any numbers you might need in an emergency.

Now put your owner's manual where you said you would and your notes where you 'think' they're going to be when you need them.

If you have any questions, call that service number you wrote down.

Accessorize To Revitalize

Keep in mind this is subjective opinion by a seasoned juicer on the must-haves, the should-have's and the maybe-later things.

If you want to make the best juice possible, you need some accessories.

Must Haves:

- Sieve for straining juices.
- Mason jars and lids.
- Measuring cups and spoons.
- Flexible rubber spatulas.
- Green produce bags.
- Kitchen scale.
- Mixing bowls – stainless steel.
- Sharp knives. If you don't have a good set of sharp knives for chopping, coring, and peeling, now's the time to invest in them.
- Cutting board. Make certain it isn't made of wood, which can transfer harmful bacteria to your juice. Replace with a heavy plastic one that is dishwasher safe.
- Cleaning Brush. On a scale of 1 to 10, this is a number 10. Brushes are indispensable for scouring all parts of your juicer. This is different from a veggie scrubber. You don't want to damage a $300 juicer with a $3 brush. They are made of nylon, brass or stainless steel.
- A stiff brush for scrubbing veggies, like carrots and beets. These brushes are cheap, but remember to be gentle, otherwise you will rub the nutritious skin off of the vegetables.
- New sponges.

• Peelers: You can go fancy, but basic works just fine. At some point down the road you might want to invest in a quality peeler removes less skin.

Accessories For Later

Now on to the accessories you might like after you have graduated to 'veteran juicer' status after a few months of juicing.

- Corers And Pitters: Handy, but hardly essential. For pineapple, a corer is great, but a good, sharp knife will work just fine.
- A sharpener for your knives
- A water filter.

And some final touches:

Salad Spinner

This helps speed up the process. You can do it by hand OR you can pop the produce into a salad spinner. Fast and simple.

The procedure is to:

1. Remove the strainer from the spinner

2. Place the lettuce or spinach into the strainer

3. Hold under the faucet to rinse thoroughly

4. Place strainer back into the spinner bowl and secure the lid

5. Turn it on or turn by hand.

Not a necessity, but it is a nice-essity (sic).

Bamboo Cutting Board

If you're 'cool,' then you better get yourself one of these. They are the hottest board out there because they are as durable as wood, yet have environmental advantages over both wood and plastic.

A grass that grows like a weed, it's 16% harder than maple.

It's unique in that harvesting doesn't kill the plant – it grows back in a few years. Hardwood, on the other hand, takes up to 60 years before it's ready to harvest. Yikes!

Biggest Plus: It has natural antimicrobial properties. When you wash a bamboo cutting board, you get extra protection because the bamboo itself kills germs.

These boards (like Hawaii tourists) also enjoy the occasional oiling.

If you are concerned about the environment and go for great quality, then I foresee bamboo in your future.

Blender

Remember way back when I said that blenders and juicers can co-exist? Now is the time to do so.

Great for extending your fresh juicing experience, creating delicious smoothies and blended soups ...Yummy.

Bigger is better with blenders, so the more you can afford, the happier you are going to be.

On a side note, Vitamix makes an amazing blender. Not sellin', just sayin'.

Price: roughly $200-800.

Dehydrator

A dehydrator is a tool that uses low temperatures to fan and dry food, removing all water from it.

I find dehydrated foods more difficult to digest, because the end products are so dry. But they are an additional food option, with good texture and certainly healthier than snacking on cookies or chips.

How do you dehydrate raw food? Simple. Just clean, cut and pop it into the dehydrator.

As long as you keep the temperature BELOW 118F, your ingredients are considered 'raw.'

How about dehydrating a smoothie? Sure, why not?

1. BLEND your favorite mix of fresh fruits and/or veggies until smooth, adding water if necessary.
2. SPREAD the mixture on a piece of cellophane, about ¼ of an inch thick.
3. PLACE the sheet in your dehydrator and dry for about 4 hours.
4. When the 'leather' is dry enough, just peel it off and flip it over to do the other side.
5. PEEL and enjoy.

Price $60-120.

Spreading Spatula

This is simply a broad, flexible, flat or offset blade knife with a round nose. It has a straight, narrow and slightly flexible nylon blade in lengths 3 ½ – 12 inches.

This makes it easy to spread or smooth toppings or mixtures and is ready for periodic scraping duties.

Price $3-10.

Zester

This is a grater, like a woodworker's rasp. It is a metal file populated by dozens of sharp teeth which cut just barely into the peel of lemons, oranges and other citrus fruits to remove just the outer edge, and shreds that into fine strips.

It can also grate nutmeg and ginger.

Price $5-8.

Sprout Bag

This is interesting. It is manufactured from industrial hemp, which is grown naturally without chemicals.

The sprout bag can grow sprouts or save them. Sprouts are expensive, so this could be a great saving. It works for all sproutable grains, nuts, vegetables seeds, beans, and gelatinous seeds.

Now pay attention, because the process is really intricate: Dip and hang. That's it.

The bags expand/contract depending on size of items inside. This is a space-saver in your refrigerator. It allows great air circulation.

Drain it without tilting. One size for ¼ cup – 2 cups. They won't break because hemp is strong, lasting for years.

Price $10-13.

Tomato Shark

This is a metal spoon which has sharp 'teeth' to dig into a strawberry or a tomato to cleanly remove the core, which leaves just fresh fruit behind.

Instead of using a knife, the tomato shark quickly eases the task.

It easy on your pocket too at $6 – $10.

Next on our docket is learning all about your choices in juicing ingredients.

4: Know Your Ingredient Types

Intro

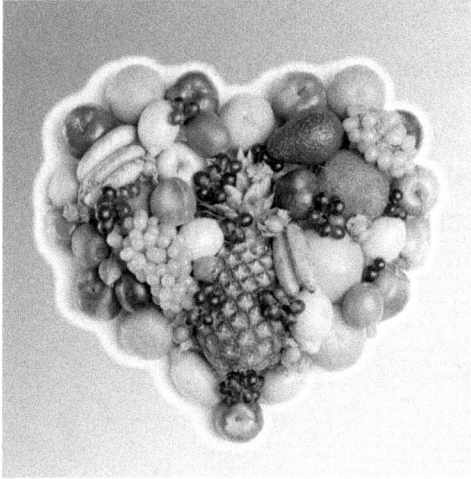

We are going to cover just *5* types of ingredients here:

1. Fruits.
2. Berries.
3. Melons
4. Spices.
5. Sweeteners.

Many other ingredient types exist, of course. Such as the magnificent greenies and veggies. They are in a league (**and a book**) of their own.

I'm starting you out with the sweeties.

Why? To develop a *taste* for juicing. If something tastes good, you are more likely to repeat. If it tastes awful, only masochists are likely to return.

Like any healthy practice, willpower will only get you so far. Then "won't power" will show you who is really in charge. If juicing is to be a significant benefit in your life, it needs to become a habit.

That is much easier achieved if you *start* with things that taste good.

Fruits are not the end point, they are the starting point. Once you learn to enjoy the taste and practice, the veggies will be waiting for you.

Fruits

Fresh fruits – they do a body good. Your body to be exact. They are filled with juicy nutrition, exactly what your body is looking for.

And when you think about fresh juice, aren't you thinking about orange, apple, or some other fruit juice?

It doesn't take a rocket scientist to deduce that orange, apple and grapefruit juice have been favorites for years. Marketing departments around the world have made sure of that.

So let's just go with it. We've been conditioned to want some color in our glass … other than green. Now green is great by me. I'm just saying let's take the path of least resistance.

We already know we like fruit juice. So let's juice some fruits. Once you taste the real deal, you will be sold. No more thin, watery, processed excuses for fruit juice. No siree, not when the real thing awaits.

Taste. That's why people love juicing.

Fresh Vegetable Juice = Yummy.

Fresh Fruit Juice = Yummy + Sweet = Yummier.

But wait, there's a downside. Welcome to life. There's always a downside.

Fresh fruit juices are high in natural sugars, so keep it reasonable in the total consumption department. Especially if you are sugar sensitive, for example, diabetics.

The "sugar spike" of all types of consumables should be considered. Generally referred to as the glycemic index, this is a number that shows the ability of a food item to increase the level of glucose in the blood.

Diabetics can address this through smaller portions or slower intake.

The juicing of veggies is certainly in your future, so fear not. After all, 'tis a lot more enjoyable to have a nice green cocktail than slog through a heaping dish of raw veggies. Again, I'm not condemning my green friends, I am merely pointing out that our journey, for now, is a sweet one.

I've gnawed many ears of corn, I've chugged thousands of gallons of glorious green goo over the years, but between you and me, a fresh and tasty glass of fruit juice ALWAYS hits the spot.

The Fiber Factor

Some people, mainly juicers, argue that plant materials, such as fruits, are inherently harder to break down. That juicing releases nutrients you would otherwise miss. Nutrients that would scoot right through your body unabsorbed.

Others say that juicing all your fruits means you'll miss out on fiber. And fiber is important because it helps with digestion and how your body handles sugars.

Guess what? Both sides have valid points.

But to turn it into an either/or situation is unnecessary. The "problem" such as it is, is quite easily fixed – just consume **some** of your fruits and vegetables whole each day. Is everybody happy now?

An apple a day ... And all that.

We'll talk more about this later.

Another way to spice things up, while getting lots of fiber is to dig out your blender from time to time. It will solve any fiber issues you might have by chopping up the fibrous pulp and mixing it with the fresh juice.

The result even has a special name – a smoothie. A yummy, healthy, fresh, fiber-filled, tasty treat.

Juicing Frequency

Some of the confusion is a result thinking of juicing as an all-or-nothing practice, like vegetarianism.

Such is not the case. There is a term for constant juicing: juice fasting. That is a very different thing and for a very different purpose.

One can be accurately referred to as a "juicer" if one on some regular basis turns produce into a liquid and consumes it. This is not a religion. There are no secret handshakes. (Well, if there are, they are still a secret to me).

My practice is to replace exactly 1 meal each day with juice. Which means, I consume 2 to 4 regular non-juiced meals each day.

Some people juice only a few times a week. Some divide the juice up into portions within a normal meal, for example having a small glass of carrot juice instead of a side dish of carrots.

See, no extremism required … or even recommended. The goal is health, not fanaticism.

Let's move on to some fun fruit facts.

Fact #1: Fruit juice does not cause obesity. Junk food and no exercise cause obesity. So don't be fooled by that great taste. Be moderate, sure. But enjoy your fruit juice.

Fact #2: Fresh strawberry juice reduces stress. Plus it tastes great. Just lean back, close your eyes, take a sip, and think … strawberry PIE. Yum.

Fact #3: Another stress buster is kiwi juice. Have you ever looked closely at a kiwi? It's a cute little brown fuzzy guy about the size of a lemon. Pick up a few the next time you're at the store.

Peel off the outer brown layer to find that they are a pretty lime green on the inside. Chop up a couple and pop into your juicer (if it has arrived) and add a couple of its fruit friends for flavoring. Kiwis alone are rather tart. But it's the effect we are after right now.

Juice it up and serve it up. Feel the stress float away (just don't try this on a Monday morning as you are rushing off to work – that would be, as we call it in the juice business, counter-productive).

Kiwi is also rich in omega 3, an amino acid that makes you smarter. And don't you feel you just made a wise choice?

Now that we've warmed up the brain cells of our imagination with fruity facts, it is time to take a really close look at a few of the workhorses of the fruit family.

You are going to be using these ingredients on a daily basis, so stock up. Fair warning.

Apples

If there were an Olympics for fruits, the apple would win the gold medal for all-around performance. It is simply the best fruit for juicing because it goes with everything. Plus it wins the award for congeniality because it is so popular. Everybody likes apples, at least they like apple juice.

Not only do people like it, but their fruit friends like it. It blends well with anything. Even those hard-to-please veggies. Because they go so well with everything, they make an excellent base.

Now for you non-chefs out there, a base is simply a liquid flavoring substance used as a basis for adding other ingredients.

Apples produce a strong juice, which makes apple juice a prime candidate for mixing with other juices.

I used to hate it when my mom sliced apples up for my school lunch, because by the time I got to them, they were more like brown mush.

You can avoid that effect by juicing a lemon just prior to apple juicing to keep the juice clear. Of course, that is only on the rare occasions when you have to make it now, but can't drink it immediately.

Apples should be stored in the refrigerator, so they keep longer. When ready for use, they should still be crisp and firm. Do not use mushy apples under the assumption that juicing will somehow "make it all better." It won't – they will still taste yucky.

What Is Good About Apples?

- Contains Vitamins A and C.
- Contains Antioxidants.
- Contains Boron – a mineral which promotes strong bones.
- Eliminates 'sleepyhead syndrome'.
- Serves up energy.
- Helps reduce bad cholesterol.
- Purges toxins from your digestive system.

- Strengthens the immune system.
- Helps digest fats.
- Full of nutrients.
- Powerful cleanser.
- General tonic for the entire system.
- Helps prevent Alzheimer's disease.
- Helps prevent cancer.

Oh, and they are reputed to keep physicians at a distance.

Cherries

Cherries are a very sweet fruit, yet they normally don't make it to the top of people's fruit lists. Perhaps it's the pits that are off-putting.

When browsing the produce section, cherries tend to get overlooked. That is a mistake. They are an excellent fruit to add to your ingredient arsenal.

Nutritional Trivia: 1 ounce of tart cherry juice concentrate has 100 calories, 1.6 g fat, 21 g carbohydrates, 21 g sugars and 0.9 g protein.

The Benefits:
- Anti-inflammatory.
- Helps relieve arthritis pain.
- Relieves joint disorders, like gout – via keracyanin.
- May help muscle recovery and reduce muscle damage.
- May inhibit tumor growth.
- Slows cardiovascular disease.
- May hinder the aging process.
- Contains flavonoids[8], anthocyanins, citric acid, malic acid and tannins.

- Contains minerals: calcium, phosphorus and potassium.
- Contains antioxidants: vitamins A, C & 13 others, including quercetin.

Grapes

Did you know there are 40 to 50 varieties of grapes?

What is your favorite color? If it is green, white, red or purple, there is a grape to match.

Danger: They should be washed thoroughly because they are highly sprayed. The white powder dust on them isn't sugar.

The stems should be green when you buy them. If a few grapes fall off the bunch, that is normal. Keep them chilled in the refrigerator until … Juice Time.

The Benefits:
- Helps reduce risk of artery blockage.
- Reduces incidence of heart attack.
- Reduces moodiness.
- Reduces depression symptoms.
- Increases 'good' cholesterol.
- Makes you smarter.
- Promotes proper alkaline blood balance.
- Stimulates kidneys.
- Regulates heartbeat.
- Cleanses the liver.
- Removes uric acid from the body.
- Contains the antioxidant quercetin.
- Contains lots of potassium.
- Contains plenty of iron.

- Contains resveratrol, which reduces heart disease (dark purple grapes).

A grape fast is reputed to lower the incidence of cancer.

Pureed seeds help make your skin look more youthful. So, inside or outside, grapes have you covered.

Grapefruit

For many people this is a morning favorite. Me, I can take 'em or leave 'em – mornings and grapefruits. But realize that there is no comparison between a fresh, juicy, organic grapefruit and a store bought one. So, if you "don't like grapefruit," give this a try, nonetheless.

Now if they would just come up with an organic morning, I'd be in business. LOL.

Most people prefer the pink over the white because it's sweeter.

You may be interested in knowing that the whitish pith in a grapefruit is excellent for you. Don't be afraid to slip a little of it into your juicer.

Did you know that grapefruit contains about 5 TIMES the amount Vitamin C as oranges? But oranges have street cred.

One final point, grapefruit can be a powerful cleanser, so don't over-do it or you'll be spending some extra "throne time," if you know what I mean.

Lemons/Limes

Just like with grapefruit, it's important to include some of the white pith from the peel when juicing these not so sweet fruits, because of the healthy bioflavinoids.

Because their juice is particularly strong, it is best to mix in other fruits, and perhaps even dilute the results of that with some water. It will definitely reduce the pucker factor.

Chilled mineral water with a splash of fresh lemon juice is especially refreshing.

Adding lemon juice to vegetable juices is another way to add variety and extra zing to what could otherwise be rather bland. Don't be afraid to experiment with your lemons and limes. Their juice is often just the spark needed to make a drink pop.

Oranges

Are you aware that frozen or bottled orange juice has virtually **no** enzymes? Don't worry though, because your drinking-from-a-bottle days are over.

Here is an interesting tidbit: Green skin on an orange does not mean it is unripe. Oranges are naturally green ... and yellow. A dye is added to the skin to make oranges ... ORANGE. Just for marketing purposes, and effective marketing it is.

Here's where my orange picking expertise comes in handy. When choosing the best oranges off the shelf, look for those with a thin and smooth skin. Heavier than you would expect is extra good because it means they are full of juice.

Valencia and Navel oranges from California are excellent for munching. While Florida oranges carry more juice.

Orange juice should be consumed faster than other juices because you are quickly losing not only enzymes, but also Vitamin C. A double loss, if you are pokey.

The Benefits:

- Powerful healing effects
- Contain a huge amount of enzymes
- Contain a huge amount of Vitamin C.

Papaya

One of the best fruits for digestion is the papaya. Adding mint to papaya juice will increase its potency, because it helps restore Vitamin C in your body.

You should **not** peel the papaya before juicing, because many of the nutrients are in the skin. However, the skin has a tendency to irritate some people. Go gentle at first with the skin to see which group you are in. You will quickly learn if you are a skin-head, so to speak.

Papaya juice is mainly carbohydrate, low in protein and fat.

Ironically, it is good for the stomach, but can **cause** stomach upset, so don't overdo it.

Nutritional Information: 1 cup contains 0.42 g protein, 0.37 g fat, and 141 calories.

The Benefits:

- Helps with digestive issues – primarily through the papain enzyme which breaks down protein.
- Helps with acid reflux and heart burn.
- Protects against cancer.
- Helps move waste products through your system.

- Natural laxative properties, helps with peristalsis.
- Contains lots of beneficial enzymes.
- Contains lots of water and soluble fiber.

Pears

I think of pears as the 'forever second' fruit. Always seeming to come in second place to that darned apple.

'A pear a day, keeps the doctor away,' just doesn't sound right. The Apple marketing folks got there first.

Ripeness is the key to pear selection. A pear is perfect when it is not too soft, nor too hard. But a hard, sour, or mushy pear is just YUCK. If anything, juicing pears should be just a little on the firm side. To get them to last for a while, keep them in your refrigerator.

Pear juice is thick and sweet, and is a prime candidate for mixing with the #1 juice (pop quiz: remember what that is?).

There is a sugar in pears, Levulose, that diabetics find especially appealing.

Bartlett, Bosc, Anjou and Comice are all popular brands, and all juice up well, if they are at the proper ripeness.

The Benefits:
- Pears have 1 advantage over apples – more pectin, for better regularity. Go pears.
- Contain great amounts of Vitamin C, calcium, potassium, phosphorus and minerals.
- Contain high levels of thiamin, riboflavin, niacin and folic acid, which aid your cardiovascular system.

Pineapples

Do you, too, think of a tropical paradise when you see a pineapple?

Taking a snooze on a cozy raft, floating worry-free amidst a warm salty breeze, enveloped by warm sunshine, needing to do absolutely nothing, palm trees swaying effortlessly in the distance, your mind saturated with nothingness.

K ... time to wake up and smell the pineapple.

Pineapples are an intimidating fruit, with their sharp, spiky leaves and their rough, hard rind, but they really are quite simple to prepare for juicing. While most people remove the rind, you can simply cut it into slices, including the core, and pop it into the juicer. It's really up to you.

When shopping, look for plump and heavy ones; the leaves should pull out easily. Dark golden color is perfect.

Store your uncut pineapples at room temperature, but the fridge is OK too.

The Benefits:
- Great for protein digestion.
- Soothes the throat.
- Can cure laryngitis.
- Helps dissolve blood clots.
- Fights cancer.
- Staves off infections.
- Keeps kidneys functioning properly – a natural diuretic.
- Contains minerals: potassium, choline, sodium, phosphorus, magnesium, sulfur, calcium, iron and iodine.
- Contains lots of vitamins, including C and bromelain.

- Contains anti-inflammatory, antiviral and antibacterial properties.
- Contains loads of nutrients and enzymes.

Tomato

That's right, a tomato is a fruit, not a vegetable, as you might think.

Why? Because it develops from the ovary of a plant. Technically speaking a tomato is classified as a berry. But because the tomato isn't as 'sweet' as most fruits, people refer to it as a vegetable.

Just some food for thought.

The red, ripe tomato is a very popular fruit for juicing. It mixes well with just about everything.

They are tasty, but turn acidic if cooked. Not that we need to care about that.

Tomato juice is very flavorful and low in calories. In case you don't like tomato sauce, that doesn't mean you won't like the juice. So give it a shot, it's a totally different animal, er plant.

The Benefits:
- Great for over-all health.
- Lowers the risk of cancer, particularly testicular.
- Great for the heart.
- Improves your immune response.
- Increases wound healing.
- Enhances iron absorption.
- Helps lower blood pressure.
- Decreases the risk of kidney stones.

- Decreases the risk of cardiovascular disease.

- Helps improve body defenses.

- Helps protect enzymes, DNA and cellular fats – where diseases usually start.

- Contains loads of minerals and vitamins.

- Contains a fine collection of potassium and vitamins E, K, C and D. Wait, we just spelled DECK. 100 points, please.

- Contains the highest percentage of lycopene of all fruits and vegetables.

OK next on the platter are sweet and delicious ...

Berries

Strawberries, blueberries, raspberries, elderberries, blackberries ... all may pop into your head when thinking of berries.

Berries are loaded with antioxidants, building up your resistance to the damaging free radicals[9] your body is constantly battling. They are also antiviral, antibacterial, and help your blood.

Berries are a bit of a nuisance to juice, but that shouldn't stop you. Pick those berries up and grind them to a pulp.

You'll find anthocyanins[2] in blackberries and blueberries ... think red wine and healthy heart.

ALL berries are nutritious, flavorful, protect against aging, help clear skin and fight cancers.

EXCEPT, the poisonous ones, so leave them alone.

Bottom line: if it looks like a berry, tastes like a berry and smells like a berry, JUICE IT!

Blackberries

Need some energy? Add blackberries to your recipes. Try it and you'll see.

Vitamin A Deficiency = Alligator Skin. Blackberries kill the alligator.

The Benefits:
- Helps keep your skin smooth and younger looking – like an Oil of Olay commercial.
- Vitamin C helps skin stay elastic (you'll be thankful after giving birth).

- Vitamin E shields skin from dangerous UV rays, thereby reduces the risk of skin cancer – 400IU a day recommended.
- Contains Vitamin A.

Black Currants

OK, now for a little background on black currants. Or Currants Events (I know, I know, I'm keeping my day job).

The black currant is the edible berry of a shrub. It's found in Northern/Central Europe and Asia. It stands 5 feet tall, the bush that is, not the berry. LOL.

The berry is about ½ inch wide, black (huh?), has a calyx at the top and a glossy skin. It also has seeds. It tastes sweet, sharp and astringent.

The Benefits:
- They are extremely high in antioxidants and vitamins.
- They contain the rare nutrients GLA and MAOI, both are used to treat depression.

So think black or you'll get blue. Speaking of which, that's our next topic.

Blueberries

Did you know you can enjoy a whole cup of blueberry for just 80 calories … and no fat?

They are loaded with Vitamin C and lots of dietary fiber.

Fiber Advantages:
- Keeps you regular.

- Helps your heart stay strong.
- Regulates "bad" cholesterol.
- Regulates sugar absorption.

The Benefits:

- Excellent antioxidant juice.
- Helps improve memory.
- Helps with urinary tract infections.
- Helps with diarrhea.
- Assists in flushing wastes from the body.
- Helps relieve menstrual cramps.
- Excellent tasting with cereal, yogurt, cottage cheese, and much more.
- Contains anthocyanins.
- Contains lots of antioxidants, including Vitamin C.
- Contains manganese – for bone development and protein conversion.

Cranberries

Suffice it to say that many people avoid these berries because they are so sour. Take note that if you combine them with apples or grapes, they juice up into a tasty treat.

Cranberries are excellent for you, but they won't win any popularity contests.

The Benefits:

- Encourages urine activity which helps with bladder issues.
- Prevents kidney stone development.
- Reduces the strong smell of urine.

- Contains virus fighting and antibiotic properties.
- Contains antioxidants aplenty.

Raspberries

Red, black, purple, gold: all are represented here. They are sweet and fruity tasting.

They are high in Vitamin C and antioxidants in general. They contain no fat, no cholesterol and no salt (shocking, I know).

Tips

Pick firm, plump, full red berries. They aren't like a banana, so won't ripen after they're picked. Ripe berries are usually deep red and will pull off the stem easily.

They cost more because they are delicate, bruising and spoiling quickly.

The Benefits:
- Keeps bacteria from populating your bladder wall.
- Reduces menstrual cramps.
- Lowers high cholesterol.
- Slows carbohydrate release (good for diabetics).
- High in fiber.
- Great source of iron and foliate, used to treat anemia.
- Has a cancer-preventing compound called ellagic acid.

Strawberries

The Benefits:
- Fiber helps digestion, decreases blood pressure, and deters overeating.

- Helps with anti-inflammatory disorders: asthma, osteoarthritis and atherosclerosis.

- Antioxidants fight many cancers.

- Decreases chances of developing macular degeneration.

- Vitamin C lowers blood pressure, improves immunity, and deters cataracts.

- Lessens cellular inflammation.

- Contains lycopene which benefits the cardiovascular system.

- Contains antioxidants from phenols.

- Contains manganese which acts as an anti-inflammatory and fights free radicals.

- Contains potassium, Vitamin K, and manganese – all great for bones.

I don't know about you, but I think this is all 'berry' good news.

We're not out of sweet stuff yet. Next up are your melons.

Melons

Cantaloupes, honey dews, watermelons: All jump to mind when I ponder the meaning of melons.

I never really thought about melons for juicing, until I tried one. I'd been missing out big time. It turns out these big guys are perfect for juicing. Sweet, juicy, and super nutritious.

The Benefits:

- High in beta carotene.
- High in folic acid.
- Loaded with Vitamins: A, B1, B2, B3, B5, B6, C, and E – a veritable alphabet soap.
- Rich in: calcium, chlorine, magnesium, phosphorus, sodium, sulfur, potassium.
- Have small amounts of: iron, copper, and zinc.
- Natural diuretics.
- Powerful cleansers.
- Excellent hydrators.
- Have antiviral and antibacterial properties.
- Contains Adenosine – an anticoagulant which helps reduce the risk of heart attack and stroke.
- Fights intestinal cancer.
- Helps with skin cancer.

A melon a day will keep the doctor away. Nice ring to that.

Cantaloupes

Cantaloupes are the most nutritious of all fruits, followed by the watermelon. Oranges acquit themselves well too. But the poor old plum is in plumb last place.

Cantaloupes have 3 times the Vitamin C of apples, and we know that apples are no slouches in that department. A lot of the nutrition is in the rind. You can juice it all, seeds and rind.

When shopping, just make sure they are neither hard nor soft, and they should have a sweet smell.

The Benefits:
- Excellent for weight loss.
- Great source of potassium – which regulates blood pressure and contracts muscles.
- Have lots of Vitamin A – for eyes, reproduction, bones, and cell division.
- Produces white cells to fight off bacteria and viruses.
- Supports the immune system.
- Creates collagen.
- Heals wounds.
- Contains the greatest amount of enzymes.

Nutritional Information: 1 serving has less than 1 g of fat and about 45 calories.

Cantaloupe definitely gets 2 thumbs up. Now how about discussing the next melon ... honey?

Honeydews

These melons are light green in color and when ripe the juicy flesh has a sweet flavor. But they take their sweet time to ripen, and meanwhile should be stored at room temperature.

The juicing process is the same as the cantaloupe: the whole thing.

The Benefits:
- Great source of vitamins A and C.
- High in potassium and zinc.
- Have lots of digestive enzymes.

And now onto those big suckers.

Watermelons

To see if it's ripe, rap it lightly with your knuckles. If there's a hollow sound, it's ready. It should be a dark green in color, with a yellow underbelly, and dull skin.

95% of the nutrients are in the rind. Although it will detract from the sweetness of the resulting juice. Try it both ways to choose your favorite.

Store them in a dry, cool place.

The Benefits:
- Helps prevent damage to DNA.
- Protects cardiovascular system.
- Helps prevent cancer.
- Cleans toxins from your system.
- Helps protect kidneys from free radical damage.
- Helps relax arteries – lowers blood pressure and increases blood flow to organs and cells.
- High water content helps flush and dissolve kidney stones.
- Helps keep bladder regular.
- Rich source of citrulline.
- Contains lycopene, an antioxidant.

- Contains lots of potassium, Vitamin C and beta-carotene.
- Contains chlorophyll, Vitamin A, protein, zinc, iodine, nucleic acids and digestive enzymes.

So you see, melons aren't just for eating. They are incredibly nutritious and great for juicing.

Moving on. Do you like it sweet or spicy?

Spices

Spicing juices improves flavor PLUS it adds valuable health benefits. Just be careful: You don't want to overpower the juice.

Universal spices for juicing: Black Pepper, Cayenne, and Turmeric.

Popular condiments: garlic, ginger, onion and parsley are awesome as veggie partners.

Black Pepper

Yup, that 'spicy' black stuff that makes you sneeze is quite popular and has lots of health benefits.

Did you know that black pepper comes from a berry? Black, green and white peppercorns are the same fruit (Piper nigrum). Why the different colors? Processing methods.

To get black pepper, you pick the pepper berries when half ripe. Leave them to dry till dark in color.

For GREEN peppercorns, pick GREEN berries.

White peppercorns are picked when ripe then soaked in brine to remove the dark shell.

Black peppers are the most pungent and flavorful of all types of peppers; they come whole, cracked, or ground.

The outermost layer of a peppercorn helps to break down fat cells. This keeps you slim, while giving you energy to burn. Very impressive.

The Benefits:
- Promotes intestinal health.
- Helps prevent gas (carminitive).
- Promotes sweating (diaphoretic).
- Promotes urination (diuretic).
- Has antibacterial and antioxidant qualities.
- Aids weight loss.
- Produces energetic feeling.
- Stimulates taste buds, increasing hydrochloric acid secretion, which aids in digestion.

Wow. Who would have thought black pepper had so many positive health benefits?

Cardamom

Has been used medicinally for thousands of years. In India, Cardamom is used for chest disorders like asthma and bronchitis.

The Benefits:
- Helps with intestinal gas and indigestion.
- Excellent tonic and pick-me-up.
- Relieves halitosis.
- Helps clear up tooth and gum disorders.
- Has diuretic properties.

Cayenne

A big source of Vitamin A, which helps cure numerous diseases.

The Benefits:
- Boosts immune system.
- Has heart benefits.
- Fights ulcers.

Cinnamon

Brings back memories of Christmas. Steaming hot cocoa with cinnamon, waiting for Santa to visit, so we could get to our presents.

OK ... back to my present ... and now back to the book.

Cinnamon grows primarily in Sri Lanka. It is taken from the bark of a type of laurel tree.

It can be purchased in stick rolls or ground up. Stick cinnamon is used to flavor liquids. Powdered is for baking.

Cinnamon is excellent for flavoring fruit juices. It has an aromatic, pleasant smell, and a sweet flavor.

The Benefits:
- Helps fight fungal infections.
- Treats gum and tooth problems.
- Prevents ulcers.
- Supports good blood sugar level.
- Helps cholesterol levels.

Ginger

Ginger is one of the most widely used herbs in the world. It's 'roots' go back at least 5,000 years. It's a rhizome, which means it has an underground stem, like bamboo.

The skin is pale tan in color and looks woody. The yellow flesh inside holds flavor, aroma and medicinal properties.

TASTE is spicy, pungent, and slightly citrus.

The Benefits:

- Anti-inflammatory and anti-viral properties.
- Fights arthritis and other inflammatory conditions.
- Helps keep your cardiovascular system healthy.
- Lowers cholesterol.
- Prevents colds.
- Is a diaphoretic.
- Acts as a digestion aid.
- Provides an energy boost
- Reduces flatulence (YUCK).
- Frequently fights flu fiercely. (OK, I'm all alliterated out now).
- Improves headaches.
- Gives your immune system a boost.
- Relieves joint pain and menstrual cramps.
- Eliminates motion sickness.
- Reduces upset stomach.

How About Juicing With Ginger?

Start with a quarter of an inch slice and peel off the outer layer. If you're tough, add some more. Put it through your juicer normally. Fresh ginger is an excellent mixer.

It may warm your fingertips a little from the volatile essential oils contained within. It can be used on the outside of the body as a stimulant.

If you have a sore throat, try some ginger and honey.

Try ginger and cantaloupe for a refreshing drink.

Nutmeg And Mace

Nutmeg and mace are similar in taste, fragrance, and actions. Both are sweet and pleasant smelling.

Nutmeg adds flavor to many juices.

Did you know that both nutmeg and mace are used for medicinal purposes?

Onions

Now it's crying time. But onions are definitely worth the tears.

The Benefits:
- Great for colds.
- Natural decongestant.
- Helps lower cholesterol.
- Contains Vitamin C.
- Excellent for boosting your immune system.
- Known as a detoxifying agent.

Turmeric

An exotic, bright yellow spice. Use just a pinch or 2 because it is potent.

The Benefits:
- Known for anti-bacterial, antibiotic and anti-inflammatory benefits.
- A detox agent with liver-cleansing properties.

Do you have a sweet tooth? I've got you covered.

Sweeteners

Agave

It's been used for many years as a natural sweetener. For taste, think raw honey and you're close.

It comes from succulents, similar to the familiar Aloe Vera for sunburns. When it's 7-10 years old, the leaves are snipped off the plant, leaving it naked. Only the core is left, which resembles a humungous pineapple (50-150 pounds). Sap is drawn from the core, filtered and warmed at low temperatures (so healthy enzymes), this process breaks down the carbohydrates into sugars.

Because low temperatures are used, it is considered a RAW FOOD. Yeah.

Agave usually comes in the form of syrup. It is quite sweet and easy to mix with liquids, even cold ones. Agave syrup comes in numerous sizes and colors, ranging from light to dark.

Agave is an excellent sweetener for raw and cooked foods.

Grape And Orange Juice

Juicing grapes makes a potent sweetener. Same with oranges, only to a lesser degree. So you are getting 2 for 1: great antioxidants plus sweetness.

Maple Syrup

Maple Syrup is usually made from the xylem sap of a sugar maple, red maple or black maple tree. It is processed by simply heating the sap, until there's only thick syrup left.

Research suggests there are more than 20 compounds in maple syrup that promote health.

The Benefits:

Several antioxidant compounds just identified in this sweet treat are also believed to:

- Help fight cancer.
- Ward off dangerous bacteria.
- Benefit diabetics.

Molasses

Think sweet tar. Molasses is made by processing sugar beets, grapes or sugar cane, converting them to sucrose. Its quality is dependent on the age of the sugar beet/cane, how much is extracted and the method used.

Sweet Sorghum Syrup = Molasses in some U.S. states ... in their heads anyway.

Technically speaking it isn't REAL molasses. Huh?

Sorghum is a crop grown for silage to feed those big black and white creatures that have horns and beautiful brown eyes.

It has an incredibly high sugar content and has been used as a sweetener for centuries.

Sorghum syrup is the most common form and you can view it in action on pancakes, cornmeal mush (YUCK), and grits. It can also replace molasses in cooking.

Raw Honey

Raw Honey is also sometimes classified as a Superfood. It will make 'Yucky' things taste yummy. It comes in several flavors.

Raw Honey by definition has not been cooked or processed. Note: There are **no** benefits to PROCESSED honey anyway.

The Benefits:
- Aids in digestion.
- Helps bronchitis.
- Has antibacterial qualities.
- Remedy for numerous healthy ailments.
- Contains antioxidants.
- Contains minerals.
- Contains amino acids.
- Contains enzymes.
- Contains carbohydrates.
- Contains phytonutrients.

Raw Sugar

Regular Sugar = Not Healthy.

Raw Sugar = Healthy (As Einstein would say, "relatively speaking").

Raw sugar has larger granules than white sugar, coarse some might say, and is a weird clear brown in color.

Stevia

Stevia is excellent for people sensitive to sugar changes, like diabetics.

Stevia Facts:

- Plant is 300 times sweeter than table sugar ... yikes.
- Glycemic index ranking of less than 1.
- Can come in liquid form.

ALERT: Stevia products are often supplemented with other sweeteners.

Sucanat

This is a brand name for various whole cane sugars. It is similar to panel and musovado because it retains its molasses content. It's really ... pure dried sugar cane juice. The juice is mechanically extracted, heated and cooled, forming small brown grainy crystals.

Costa Rica is where it lives, but it is repackaged in the United States.

Unlike traditional brown sugar, vitamins, minerals and molasses are not displaced during the processing. That's great news.

Yams And Bananas

Cooked yams and bananas are sweet. It's easy to puree them to increase the sweetness even more.

Both add flavor and trace amounts of minerals and fiber for bonus points.

Sugar Types (There are many variations on this sweet theme)

Glucose

Simple sugar is made when the body digests carbohydrates. This is actually the primary energy source for the whole body. Scary.

Another common name is dextrose.

Sucrose

This is your normal everyday table sugar. It comes from sugar beets or sugar cane and it is highly processed. And that is not a good thing. It is a combination of 2 other sugars: fructose and glucose, but during digestion they separate back to their native forms.

It is very sweet and would be perfect, except for 2 tiny little flaws: it is not healthy and has no nutrients whatsoever. Other than that, it's fine.

Fructose

Often called fruit sugar, fructose comes from tree fruits, honey, melons, and berries. Its crystalline form is from sucrose (see above) or corn.

To produce it, you hydrolyze sucrose or process corn starch (respectively). Either way, a heap of processing going on.

High Fructose Syrup

This comes from corn, wheat or rice starches and is virtually identical to our old friend, sucrose. Due to governmental intervention, it is cheap, so it's found in lots of 'Yucky' processed foods.

Fructose is 50% sweeter than sucrose, but its glycemic index is thankfully low. However, don't think that lets you off the hook. Since the liver must process it, too much at once will still get you into trouble.

The liver will turn the excess into triglycerides, which can cause cells to become resistant to insulin. That leads to diabetes and cholesterol increases. All that for NO nutrition.

Maltose

Malt sugar is made from the starches of wheat, barley, rice and other grains. It's only half the sweetness of sucrose and it is used for making beer.

In your body maltose is the first stage of digesting starches, which are later reduced to glucose.

Lactose

Sugar specific to milk is referred to as lactose. As in the ever-growing trend of "lactose intolerant."

Date Sugar

To manufacture date sugar, dehydrated dates are chewed into tiny pieces. Mechanically, not by dogs. Most health practitioners give it a thumbs up as a sugar substitute.

- High in fiber.
- Lots of vitamins.
- High in minerals.

Recap

Just remember, when you HAVE to have a little more sweetness in your juice de jour, instead of nasty old sugar, reach for one of these:

Agave, bananas, dates, chopped figs, grape juice, raw honey, maltose, maple syrup, molasses, raisins, Stevia, or yams.

With all these choices, you have no excuse to pig out on white sugar any longer.

And when you want to spice up your juice:

Celery seed, cinnamon, ginger, mace, nutmeg, onions, one of the peppers (but not the Doctor), or turmeric.

These spices increase the possible combinations astronomically, making it difficult to get bored with even a few recipes.

But wait, you have even more combination options coming up.

Oran Kangas

5: How To Avoid Juice Boredom

Intro

This chapter will deal with final matters to get you ready for a lifetime of juicing.

3 ways of avoiding juicing boredom are examined:

1. Substitutions.
2. Smoothies (yes, they are not the enemy).
3. Recycling pulp.

Finally a section on naming.

Then it's off to Juice Recipe heaven.

Bring In The Substitutes

One problem with any dietary activity that one is considering to adopt for a lifetime, is boredom. Sure there are many recipes that taste great. But are there a lifetime worth of them?

You can buy several juicing recipe books to handle that problem, or you can simply make some judicious substitutions. Any substitute will greatly affect the flavor, lending a huge boost to the number of combinations possible.

Another fine tuning approach is to vary the amount of an ingredient. Again a wealth of more subtle flavor shifts are presented.

What are these *magical* substitutes?

- **Pineapple, apple, and orange** >> work well for replacing almost any fruit.

- **Lime** >> for any citrus.

- **Carrot** >> for a veggie.

- **Romaine lettuce** >> for a greenie.

- **Cinnamon** >> for ginger.

But guess what? Those 5 subs are not at all magical. Almost any item will stand in for a family member: a fruit for any fruit, etc. I am speaking of nutrition here.

Taste-wise, it might be a disaster. So substitute cautiously. It is usually a good idea to cut the quantity of an unknown sub in half first round. Trial and error is the order of the day.

Juicing needs never get boring.

Smoothies

Don't forget to try an occasional smoothie. It is quite a bit like a juice, in fact you can often use precisely the same recipes and get a different taste sensation.

Note: Smoothies should be made in a different machine – a blender, because a juicer thins it out by extracting all the pulp. Which is exactly what we want in juicing.

Smoothies have a thicker consistency, more like a milkshake.

One definite advantage a smoothie has over a juice is more **fiber**, which helps with elimination and many other things.

Another neat trick is to toss in some exotic ingredients, like chocolate, peanut butter, yogurt, ice-cream, whey powder, protein powder, green tea, herbal supplements, nutritional supplements, crushed ice, etc.

You might as well grab some gooey items that just will not juice properly as you walk on the wild side.

Frozen Treats

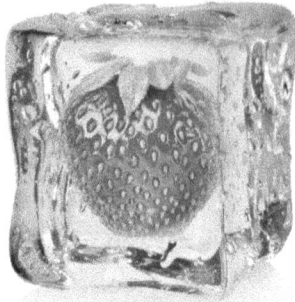

When it comes to juicing you're going to end up with loads of PULP. What to do, what to do? Waste Not, Want Not.

We know pulp is LOADED with fiber. So we have 2 options:

1. Chuck it. (Into the compost, of course).
2. Or ... eat it.

If you choose to eat it, you have 3 temperature zones:

1. Hot – cook with it.
2. Medium – re-juice it.
3. Cold – make frozen treats.

Cooking destroys enzymes, we have already discussed juicing ad nauseum, so it's time to enter the cold zone.

Frozen Treat Popsicles

The pulp from your fresh juices is an excellent way to get fiber and vital nutrients into something tasty and fun. Berry juice pulp is especially superb for popsicles.

Here's another recipe: add yogurt and some honey to your pulp.

Method:

1. Add water to some fresh or thawed pulp.
2. Pour the mixture into an ice cube tray.
3. Put Cling Wrap over the tray.
4. Poke a stick in the middle of each slot.
5. Place the ice tray into the freezer compartment.

In just a few hours, you'll have your own home-made popsicles.

Frozen Treat Drinks

I suggest that you place your pulp in freezer bags, and lay them out flat on a freezer shelf. When needed, you can easily break off just the right amount.

You can prepare your favorite juice or smoothie recipe by substituting the frozen pulp for 1 or 2 of the ingredients. Then pop the results into your juicing machine.

Presto, you will have a fiber-filled flavorful favorite. Say that fast 3 times.

The Name Game

Often authors simply slap a silly name on their concoction, for example "The Miami Heat Cooler." What is the point?

That name means nothing, conveys nothing, and should you ever try to use it even with a fellow juicer, you will get nothing but a blank stare.

Instead of that, I will be using a less creative, but more helpful naming system. It looks a bit like some strange form of 'juicing math.'

oranges + grapefruits + lemons = Orange-Grapefruit-Lemon Juice

The *ingredients* on the left produce the *drink* on the right side. Or in reverse, if you know the name, you instantly know the ingredients.

One more fine point, we take the ingredients roughly in order of their size to name the drink.

So, in the above example, we know that oranges are the main item, grapefruits are secondary (or possibly equal in mass), and lemons are likely a bit player.

Now that you know everything, let's get to the meat of the matter. Real fruit juice recipes. Starting with ... The Miami Heat Cooler. ☺

PART 3: FRUIT JUICE RECIPES

Intro

Now we are into the cream of the crop. You have officially arrived at the Good Stuff.

So exciting!

Only 2 chapters, but they are whoppers:

1. 30 Recipes.
2. Nutritional values within those recipes.

Oran Kangas

6: Getting It Together – 30 Recipes For Success

Sizing

But before we get started, we should clear up some confusion surrounding the amount of juice you should make. Many authors leave unclear what their sizing standards are. So you might make 1 recipe and it won't even fill a glass. Make the next and it serves an Army. Some standards, please.

The 3 main measurements we repeatedly came across in the literature are:

Portion size, Serving size, and Meal replacement size.

To be clear, I will be using a 16 ounce serving of juice as the standard, which is the equivalent of a FULL MEAL REPLACEMENT for 1 person. So, every recipe presented from here on is designed to be a meal for 1.

You can adjust a little more or less, depending on your size, weight and muscle to fat ratio, if you want to more precise. Men generally get more juice and women less. In actuality, gender doesn't matter. Body composition is what is important, technically speaking.

If you just want to use juicing as a side dish, say carrot juice instead of carrots, divide the given recipe by 3. Clear?

This will explain the sticker shock when you see the calorie count.

Customization Plan

Since everyone's tastes are different, you should be prepared to make some minor modifications to the recipes. I call it the customization plan. You should get a notepad, anything will do. Just take it a notch above random scraps of paper, okay?

Follow a recipe, then record in your notebook the recipe number and ANY changes you made this time or want to try out next time.

Repeat the process with every juicing. You'll soon have a notebook filled with custom recipes, fine-tuned just for your taste buds.

Pay attention now. I just gave you **the Secret Sauce!**

With a little tinkering, you can now turn nearly anything into something you actually enjoy. That is power. You are no longer at the mercy of the "recipe maker," hoping she came up with something you like. You can MAKE it something you like.

Or at least come to a realization that (like a certain former President) you HATE broccoli (or whatever your culinary adversary is). Learn to love it or learn to substitute for it.

This is important! This is very, very important! So important that I will remind you on each recipe with the following message:

[Record any changes you'd like to try next time in your Customization Notebook]

Getting Started

OK ... Now that we've gotten that straightened out, let's give you a TASTE of your first recipe.

Time for you to get wet in the Wonderful World Of Juicing, to enjoy the fruits of your labor (sorry).

If you have not yet ordered your juicer, (OMG why not?) it's time to pick up the phone.

And 1 last thing before I turn you loose into the wilds of recipe land, locate an organic source of fresh fruits and vegetables.

If you're in it for the health of it, go organic.

Recipe #1:
Apple–Pineapple–Ginger Juice

CALORIES: 316 (16 oz. serving – Meal Replacement for 1)

FOR: Antioxidants and high vitamin count are good for almost everything.

INGREDIENTS:

2 Apples

2 cups Pineapple

½ tsp. Ginger (Fresh)

PREPARATION: [5 minutes]

Wash all ingredients.

Cut apple into chunks with skin on; remove seeds.

Remove pineapple rind (or not), cut into chunks.

Place all ingredients into machine.

Hit Start.

Add 1 cup ice to your glass (optional)

**[Record any changes you'd like to try next time in your
Customization Notebook]**

FINAL WARNING: Seriously, folks, this is the most important step of all. No recipe from *any* source will taste "right" for everybody. If you don't make micro-changes for your palate, you are cheating yourself of flavor. And probably undermining your entire health change program.

Recipe #2:
Apple–Strawberry–Blueberry–Raspberry Juice

CALORIES: 143 (16 oz. serving – Meal Replacement for 1)

FOR: Many claims can be and are made. That the individual ingredients are healthy and health-promoting I stand behind. That 1 particular "magical" blend will cure any exact illness, I can no longer support. There just does not exist enough evidence on this micro level.

This is a departure from the first edition of this book. For entertainment purposes, I have moved that data to the next chapter (Nutritional Values).

INGREDIENTS:

1 Apple

½ cup Strawberries

¼ cup Blueberries

¼ cup Raspberries

PREPARATION: [5 minutes]

Wash all ingredients.

Cut apple into chunks with skin on; remove seeds.

Top strawberries.

Place all ingredients into machine.

Hit Start.

Add 1 cup ice to your glass (optional).

[Record any changes you'd like to try next time in your Customization Notebook]

Recipe #3:
Apple-Strawberry-Grape Juice

CALORIES: 271 (16 oz. serving – Meal Replacement for 1)

INGREDIENTS:

2 Apples

1 cup Strawberries

1 cup Grapes

PREPARATION: [5 minutes]

Wash all ingredients.

Cut apple into chunks with skin on; remove seeds.

Place all ingredients into machine.

Hit Start.

Add 1 cup ice to your glass (optional).

[Record any changes you'd like to try next time in your Customization Notebook]

Oran Kangas

The Pause Button

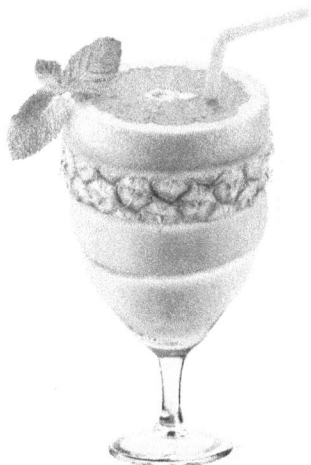

It's Time For Reflection

We are past the hump, into the home stretch, on the downhill slope, and sliding into home. Did I overlook any metaphorical clichés?

Whatever, you can clearly see where we've been and where we are going. There's lots of *stuff* ahead, of course, but our *course* is clear.

Is it time to celebrate, as the graphic above implies? Or are you uneasy about something?

Is the picture becoming clear, and revealing a future of juicing ahead for you? Or is the prognosis murky or worse.

This is a critical point in the book for many people. Speaking in the abstract, since I don't know you personally, I nonetheless know that a significant number of people unconsciously give up on a book, any book, when they reach a certain stage. I call it the "Are We There Yet?" Stage.

Such folks (and that's everybody from time to time, myself included) enter a book with high hopes. This is the book that will change my life! We are too sophisticated to say that out loud, but still the hope, the dream is there as we click the Buy button.

Until now you have patiently sat through the theory of this book, knowing that when you got to the recipes ... that would be *it!*

Well, is it?

Unlikely. You have had 3 recipes to sample and the world has probably not taken a dramatic change for the better. If it has ... Hallelujah! Pass me whatever you are drinking!

The sad, sad truth is that significant change takes significant time. If our hopes are too high and our timeline too short, disappointment is almost inevitable.

Let's do a quick assessment before we trudge on toward Nirvana.

There is a Glossary at the back with hyperlinks explaining all the difficult terms from the early chapters. Remember my suggestion that you follow them? Did you? Hmmm. Way back there some of you made a decision. To quit.

I will wager that there is a similar pattern: in your reading, career, and life. You approach change, then draw back. Hope, then withdraw hope, to avoid disappointment.

Juicing will not affect that one way or the other. But self-awareness will.

Your life, your call.

A final check, if you will indulge me. I have virtually pleaded with you to create a recipe customization log. I have explained why. I have reminded you on every recipe.

Let's have a show of hands: did you do it? If not, w-h-y?

If you think I am beating a dead horse here, it is because I am trying to restore it to life.

It is my belief that an author, every author, has a duty to try to make each reader's life better. Should the reader not share that goal for him/herself?

If anyone feels insulted, please know that is not my intent. Nor is it personal. How could it be? I've never seen you, and likely never will.

I shall put away the soap box now.

It's time to mellow out with some heavy drinking. Juiced, of course.

Recipe #4:
Apple–Cucumber–Ginger Juice

CALORIES: 267 (16 oz. serving – Meal Replacement for 1)

INGREDIENTS:

3 Apples

½ Cucumber

2 tsp. Ginger (Fresh)

PREPARATION: [5 minutes]

Wash all ingredients.

Cut apple into chunks with skin on; remove seeds.

Cut the other ingredients to fit into machine.

Place all ingredients into machine.

Hit Start.

Add 1 cup ice to your glass (optional).

**[Record any changes you'd like to try next time in your
Customization Notebook]**

Recipe #5:
Apple–Grape–Lemon Juice

CALORIES: 527 (16 oz. serving – Meal Replacement for 1)

INGREDIENTS:

5 Apples

2 cups Grapes

1/8 Lemon

PREPARATION: [5 minutes]

Wash all ingredients.

Cut apples into chunks with skin on; remove seeds.

Peel lemon rind, leaving some white pith.

Place ingredients into machine.

Hit Start.

Add 1 cup ice to your glass (optional).

[Record any changes you'd like to try next time in your
Customization Notebook]

Recipe #6:
Apple–Kiwi–Blackberry Juice

FOR: Vitamins and antioxidants

CALORIES: 387 (16 oz. serving – Meal Replacement for 1)

INGREDIENTS:

2 Apples

1 Kiwi

1 cup Blackberries

1 cup Seltzer Water

1 tsp. Agave (sweeten to taste)

PREPARATION: [5 minutes]

Wash all ingredients.

Cut apple into chunks with skin on; remove seeds.

Peel kiwis.

Cut all ingredients to fit into machine.

Place all ingredients into machine.

Hit Start.

Add 1 cup ice to your glass (optional).

[Record any changes you'd like to try next time in your Customization Notebook]

Recipe #7:
Apple–Lemon–Ginger Juice

CALORIES: 263 (16 oz. serving – Meal Replacement for 1)

INGREDIENTS:

3 Apples

½ Lemon

1 tsp. Ginger (Fresh)

PREPARATION: [5 minutes]

Wash all ingredients.

Cut apple into chunks with skin on; remove seeds.

Peel lemon rind, leaving some white pith.

Cut all ingredients to fit into machine.

Place all ingredients into machine.

Hit Start.

Add 1 cup ice to your glass (optional).

[Record any changes you'd like to try next time in your
Customization Notebook]

Recipe #8:
Apple–Orange–Pear–Lemon Juice

CALORIES: 323 (16 oz. serving – Meal Replacement for 1)

INGREDIENTS:

2 Apples

1 Orange

1 Pear

1 slice Lemon

PREPARATION: [5 minutes]

Wash all ingredients.

Peal orange.

Peel lemon rind, leaving some white pith.

Remove pear and apple stems.

Cut ingredients to fit into machine.

Put all ingredients in machine.

Hit Start.

Add 1 cup ice to your glass (optional).

[Record any changes you'd like to try next time in your Customization Notebook]

Recipe #9:
Apple–Raspberry–Orange–Spirulina Juice

CALORIES: 346 (16 oz. serving – Meal Replacement for 1)

INGREDIENTS:

2 Apples

2 cups of Raspberries

1 Orange

1 tsp. Spirulina (optional)

PREPARATION: [5 minutes]

Wash all ingredients.

Cut apples into chunks with skin on; remove seeds.

Peel orange.

Cut all ingredients to fit into machine.

Place all ingredients into machine.

Hit Start.

Pour the juice into a container with a lid.

Add the Spirulina, close the lid, and shake vigorously.

Add 1 cup ice to your glass (optional).

**[Record any changes you'd like to try next time in your
Customization Notebook]**

Recipe #10:
Apple–Strawberry–Banana Juice

CALORIES: 294 (16 oz. serving – Meal Replacement for 1)

INGREDIENTS:

2 Apples

½ cup Strawberries

1 Banana

1 tsp. Stevia (sweeten to taste)

PREPARATION: [5 minutes]

Wash all ingredients.

Cut apples into chunks with skin on; remove seeds.

Place all ingredients into machine.

Hit Start.

Add 1 cup ice to your glass (optional).

[Record any changes you'd like to try next time in your Customization Notebook]

Recipe #11:
Blackberry–Raspberry–Strawberry Juice

CALORIES: 294 (16 oz. serving – Meal Replacement for 1)

INGREDIENTS

¼ cup Blackberries

¼ cup Raspberries

¼ cup Strawberries

2 cups Seltzer Water

1 tbsp. Agave (sweeten to taste)

PREPARATION: [5 minutes]

Wash all ingredients.

Top strawberries.

Place all ingredients in machine.

Hit Start.

Add 1 cup ice to your glass (optional).

[Record any changes you'd like to try next time in your
Customization Notebook]

Recipe #12:
Blueberry–Blackberry–Strawberry–Grape –Lemon Juice

CALORIES: 263 (16 oz. serving – Meal Replacement for 1)

INGREDIENTS

1 cup Blueberries

1 cup Blackberries

1 cup Strawberries

1 cup Grapes

½ Lemon

PREPARATION: [5 minutes]

Wash all ingredients.

Top strawberries.

Peel lemon rind, leaving some white pith.

Cut ingredients to fit into machine.

Place all ingredients in machine.

Hit Start.

Add 1 cup ice to your glass (optional).

[Record any changes you'd like to try next time in your Customization Notebook]

Recipe #13:
Blueberry–Kiwi Juice

CALORIES: 545 (16 oz. serving – Meal Replacement for 1)

INGREDIENTS:

5 Cups Blueberries

3 Kiwis

PREPARATION: [5 minutes]

Wash all ingredients.

Peel Kiwis.

Place all ingredients in machine.

Hit Start.

Add 1 cup ice to your glass (optional).

[Record any changes you'd like to try next time in your Customization Notebook]

Recipe #14:
Currant–Pineapple Juice

CALORIES: 296 (16 oz. serving – Meal Replacement for 1)

INGREDIENTS:

2 cups Currants

2 cups Pineapple

1 pinch Cinnamon

PREPARATION: [5 minutes]

Remove pineapple rind (or not).

Cut ingredients to fit into your machine.

Put all ingredients into your machine.

Hit Start.

Add 1 cup ice to your glass (optional).

[Record any changes you'd like to try next time in your Customization Notebook]

Recipe #15:
Grapefruit–Papaya Juice

CALORIES: 360 (16 oz. serving – Meal Replacement for 1)

INGREDIENTS:

1 Grapefruit

2 cups Papaya

PREPARATION: [5 minutes]

Wash all ingredients.

Peel grapefruit.

Cut fruit to fit into your machine.

Place all ingredients in machine.

Hit Start.

Add 1 cup ice to your glass (optional).

[Record any changes you'd like to try next time in your Customization Notebook]

Recipe #16:
Melon–Apple–Pear–Lemon Juice

CALORIES: 392 (16 oz. serving – Meal Replacement for 1)

INGREDIENTS:

½ Honeydew Melon

2 Apples

1 Pear

½ Lemon

A few Mint leaves

PREPARATION: [5 minutes]

Wash all ingredients.

Cut apples into chunks with skin on; remove seeds.

Peel lemon rind, leaving some white pith.

Cut ingredients to fit into your machine.

Place all ingredients in machine.

Hit Start.

Add 1 cup ice to your glass (optional).

[Record any changes you'd like to try next time in your Customization Notebook]

Oran Kangas

Recipe #17:
Orange–Apple–Raspberry–Strawberry Juice

CALORIES: 278 (16 oz. serving – Meal Replacement for 1)

INGREDIENTS:

1 Orange

2 Apples

½ cup Raspberries

½ cup Strawberries

PREPARATION: [5 minutes]

Wash all ingredients.

Cut apples into chunks with skin on; remove seeds.

Peel oranges.

Cut all ingredients to fit into machine.

Place ingredients into machine.

Hit Start.

Add 1 cup ice to your glass (optional).

[Record any changes you'd like to try next time in your Customization Notebook]

Recipe #18:
Orange–Carrot–Cinnamon Juice

CALORIES: 198 (16 oz. serving – Meal Replacement for 1)

INGREDIENTS:

2 Oranges

3 Carrots

1 dash cinnamon

PREPARATION: [5 minutes]

Wash all ingredients.

Peel orange.

Cut all ingredients to fit into machine.

Place ingredients into machine.

Hit Start.

Add 1 cup ice to your glass (optional).

[Record any changes you'd like to try next time in your Customization Notebook]

Recipe #19:
Orange–Grapefruit–Lemon Juice

CALORIES: 270 (16 oz. serving – Meal Replacement for 1)

INGREDIENTS:

4 Oranges

¼ Grapefruit

¼ Lemon

PREPARATION: [5 minutes]

Wash all ingredients.

Peel oranges.

Peel lemon rind, leaving some white pith.

Peel grapefruit.

Cut all ingredients to fit into machine.

Place ingredients into machine.

Hit Start.

Add 1 cup ice to your glass (optional).

**[Record any changes you'd like to try next time in your
Customization Notebook]**

Recipe #20:
Pineapple–Grape–Ginger Juice

CALORIES: 351 (16 oz. serving – Meal Replacement for 1)

INGREDIENTS:

3 cups Pineapple

2 cups Grapes

1 tsp. Ginger

1 cup Sparkling Water

PREPARATION: [5 minutes]

Wash all ingredients.

Remove pineapple rind (or not).

Cut all ingredients to fit into machine.

Place ingredients into machine.

Hit Start.

Mix Sparkling Water with juice when finished.

Add 1 cup ice to your glass (optional).

[Record any changes you'd like to try next time in your Customization Notebook]

Recipe #21:
Pineapple–Orange–Grape–Strawberry Juice

CALORIES: 288 (16 oz. serving – Meal Replacement for 1)

INGREDIENTS:

2 cups Pineapple

1 Orange

1 cup Grapes

1/3 cup Strawberries

PREPARATION: [5 minutes]

Wash all ingredients

Remove pineapple rind (or not).

Peel orange.

Top strawberries.

Cut all ingredients to fit into machine.

Place all ingredients into machine.

Hit Start.

Add 1 cup ice to your glass (optional).

[Record any changes you'd like to try next time in your Customization Notebook]

Recipe #22:
Pineapple–Orange–Lime Juice

CALORIES: 267 (16 oz. serving – Meal Replacement for 1)

INGREDIENTS:

¼ Pineapple

1 Orange

1/8 Lime

PREPARATION: [5 minutes]

Wash all ingredients

Remove pineapple rind (or not).

Peel oranges and lime.

Cut all ingredients to fit into machine.

Place all ingredients in machine.

Hit Start.

Add 1 cup ice to your glass (optional).

**[Record any changes you'd like to try next time in your
Customization Notebook]**

Recipe #23:
Pineapple–Papaya–Kiwi Juice

CALORIES: 338 (16 oz. serving – Meal Replacement for 1)

INGREDIENTS:

3 cups Pineapple

½ Papaya

1 Kiwi

PREPARATION: [5 minutes]

Wash all ingredients

Remove pineapple rind (or not).

Peel Kiwi.

Remove seed from papaya.

Cut all ingredients to fit into machine.

Place all ingredients in machine.

Hit Start.

Add 1 cup ice to your glass (optional).

[Record any changes you'd like to try next time in your
Customization Notebook]

Recipe #24:
Plum–Orange–Ginger Juice

CALORIES: 428 (16 oz. serving – Meal Replacement for 1)

INGREDIENTS:

12 Plums

1 Orange

1 tsp. Ginger

PREPARATION: [5 minutes]

Wash all ingredients.

Peel orange.

Cut all ingredients to fit into machine.

Place all ingredients into machine.

Hit Start.

Add 1 cup ice to your glass (optional).

[Record any changes you'd like to try next time in your Customization Notebook]

Recipe #25:
Strawberry–Blueberry–Raspberry Juice

CALORIES: 187 (16 oz. serving – Meal Replacement for 1)

INGREDIENTS:

1 cup Strawberries

1 cup Blueberries

1 cup Raspberries

PREPARATION: [5 minutes]

Wash all ingredients.

Top strawberries.

Cut all ingredients to fit into machine.

Place ingredients into machine.

Hit Start.

Add 1 cup ice to your glass (optional).

[Record any changes you'd like to try next time in your
Customization Notebook]

Recipe #26:
Watermelon–Honeydew–Cantaloupe Juice

CALORIES: 1,277 (16 oz. serving – Meal Replacement for 1)

INGREDIENTS:

½ Watermelon

1 Honeydew Melon

1 Cantaloupe

PREPARATION: [5 minutes]

Wash all ingredients.

Remove all rinds (or not).

Cut melons to fit into the machine.

Place all ingredients into machine.

Hit Start.

Add 1 cup ice to your glass (optional).

[Record any changes you'd like to try next time in your Customization Notebook]

Recipe #27:
Watermelon–Lemon Juice

FOR: Cooler, hydration

CALORIES: 384 (16 oz. serving – Meal Replacement for 1)

INGREDIENTS:

¼ Watermelon

1 Lemon

PREPARATION: [5 minutes]

Wash all ingredients.

Remove watermelon rind (or not).

Peel lemon rind, leaving some white pith.

Cut all ingredients to fit into machine.

Place ingredients into machine

Hit Start.

Add 1 cup ice to your glass (optional).

[Record any changes you'd like to try next time in your
Customization Notebook]

Recipe #28:
Watermelon–Orange–Mango–Pineapple–Strawberry Juice

CALORIES: 404 (16 oz. serving – Meal Replacement for 1)

INGREDIENTS:

4 cups Watermelon

1 Orange

½ Mango

½ cup Pineapple

6 Strawberries

PREPARATION: [5 minutes]

Wash all ingredients.

Remove pineapple and watermelon rinds (or not).

Peel orange.

Top strawberries.

Cut all ingredients to fit into machine.

Place all ingredients into machine.

Hit Start.

Add 1 cup ice to your glass (optional).

[Record any changes you'd like to try next time in your
Customization Notebook]

Recipe #29:
Watermelon–Orange–Pineapple–Lemon Juice

CALORIES: 1,096 (16 oz. serving – Meal Replacement for 1)

INGREDIENTS:

½ Watermelon

6 Oranges

2 cups Pineapple

1 Lemon

PREPARATION: [5 minutes]

Wash all ingredients.

Peel lemon rind, leaving some white pith.

Remove watermelon rind (or not).

Cut all ingredients to fit into machine.

Place ingredients into machine.

Hit Start.

Add 1 cup ice to your glass (optional).

[Record any changes you'd like to try next time in your Customization Notebook]

Recipe #30:
Watermelon–Pineapple–Orange–Kiwi–Lemon Juice

CALORIES: 1,246 (16 oz. serving – Meal Replacement for 1)

INGREDIENTS:

½ Watermelon

½ Pineapple

4 Oranges

2 Kiwis

1 Lemon

PREPARATION: [5 minutes]

Wash all ingredients.

Peel lemon rind, leaving some white pith.

Remove watermelon & pineapple rinds (or not).

Peel oranges and kiwis.

Cut all ingredients to fit into machine.

Place ingredients into machine.

Hit Start.

Add 1 cup ice to your glass (optional).

[Record any changes you'd like to try next time in your Customization Notebook]

7: Nutritional Values Of The 30 Juicing Recipes

Now you have some solid recipes to choose from. Perhaps you would like to know a little more about what is in each of them. Perhaps you want to know a LOT about that. This chapter has you covered.

Each recipe is presented here in order. You will likely find more than you ever wanted to know here. Or you can just skip this chapter entirely. Your call.

All the following Daily Value percentages are based on an assumed 2,000 calorie diet. Since yours is likely less than that, you can make the necessary adjustments in your head ... or use a calculator if you want to be all exact about it.

To skip ahead to the next chapter, turn to page 185.

Recipe #1:
Apple–Pineapple–Ginger

Total Fat 1.8g

Saturated Fat 0.2g

Polyunsaturated Fat 0.6g

Monounsaturated Fat 0.2g

Cholesterol 0.0mg

Sodium 3.4mg

Potassium 672.2mg

Total Carbohydrate 80.8g

Dietary Fiber 11.4g

Sugars 59.6g

Protein 1.6g

Vitamin A 4.2%

Vitamin B-12 0.0%

Vitamin B-6 20.1%

Vitamin C 105.9%

Vitamin D 0.0%

Vitamin E 6.0%

Calcium 4.2%

Copper 22.9%

Folate 10.7%

Iron 9.3%

Magnesium 14.5%

Manganese 261.9%

Niacin 7.9%

Pantothenic Acid 6.8%

Phosphorus 4.3%

Riboflavin 8.8%

Selenium 3.8%

Thiamin 22.2%

Zinc 2.2%

Recipe #2:
Apple–Blueberry–Strawberry– Raspberry

Claimed to be "FOR: Anti-cancer & anti-heart disease benefits, plus it may reduce "bad" cholesterol"

Total Fat 0.7g	Vitamin D 0.0%
Saturated Fat 0.1g	Vitamin E 5.2%
Polyunsaturated Fat 0.4g	Calcium 2.9%
Monounsaturated Fat 0.1g	Copper 6.8%
Cholesterol 0.0mg	Folate 6.8%
Sodium 2.9mg	Iron 4.2%
Potassium 357.3mg	Magnesium 5.4%
Total Carbohydrate 34.8g	Manganese 34.2%
Dietary Fiber 8.5g	Niacin 3.4%
Sugars 21.4g	Pantothenic Acid 4.4%
Protein 1.2g	Phosphorus 3.1%
Vitamin A 3.3%	Riboflavin 6.6%
Vitamin B-12 0.0%	Selenium 1.9%
Vitamin B-6 6.9%	Thiamin 4.3%
Vitamin C 101.8%	Zinc 2.1%

Recipe #3:
Apple–Strawberry–Grape

Claimed to be "FOR: Colds"

Total Fat 1.9g	Vitamin D 0.0%
Saturated Fat 0.5g	Vitamin E 11.1%
Polyunsaturated Fat 0.8g	Calcium 5.9%
Monounsaturated Fat 0.1g	Copper 16.7%
Cholesterol 0.0mg	Folate 10.4%
Sodium 4.7mg	Iron 8.4%
Potassium 745.8mg	Magnesium 9.7%
Total Carbohydrate 68.9g	Manganese 32.8%
Dietary Fiber 11.8g	Niacin 5.2%
Sugars 50.6g	Pantothenic Acid 7.4%
Protein 1.8g	Phosphorus 7.0%
Vitamin A 6.0%	Riboflavin 13.5%
Vitamin B12 20.0%	Selenium 3.1%
Vitamin B6 19.9%	Thiamin 15.0%
Vitamin C 198.7%	Zinc 2.5%

Recipe #4:
Apple–Cucumber–Ginger

Claimed to be "FOR: joint pain"

Total Fat 0.8g	Vitamin D 0.0%
Saturated Fat 0.4g	Vitamin E 7.0%
Polyunsaturated Fat 0.4g	Calcium 3.9%
Monounsaturated Fat 0.0g	Copper 10.8%
Cholesterol 0.0mg	Folate 5.0%
Sodium 2.5mg	Iron 5.4%
Potassium 596.8mg	Magnesium 7.9%
Total Carbohydrate 66.6g	Manganese 12.6%
Dietary Fiber 11.9g	Niacin 2.6%
Sugars 41.6g	Pantothenic Acid 3.8%
Protein 1.2g	Phosphorus 4.4%
Vitamin A 6.5%	Riboflavin 4.3%
Vitamin B12 20.0%	Selenium 1.8%
Vitamin B6 11.9%	Thiamin 5.7%
Vitamin C 44.9%	Zinc 1.9%

Recipe #5:
Apple–Grape–Lemon

Claimed to be "FOR: Constipation, indigestion, fatigue, kidney disorders, macular degeneration, cataracts, slow aging, asthma, heart disease. Migraine: home remedy, take early in the morning"

Total Fat 1.6g

Saturated Fat 1.1g

Polyunsaturated Fat 1.1g

Monounsaturated Fat 0.0g

Cholesterol 0.0mg

Sodium 6.2mg

Potassium 1,132.8mg

Total Carbohydrate 136.3g

Dietary Fiber 20.6g

Sugars 97.8g

Protein 2.0g

Vitamin A 11.4%

Vitamin B12 0.0%

Vitamin B6 33.5%

Vitamin C 120.9%

Vitamin D 0.0%

Vitamin E 21.8%

Calcium 8.4%

Copper 28.3%

Folate 8.0%

Iron 11.4%

Magnesium 13.6%

Manganese 24.5%

Niacin 7.6%

Pantothenic Acid 5.3%

Phosphorus 9.0%

Riboflavin 15.9%

Selenium 4.0%

Thiamin 26.8%

Zinc 2.5%

Recipe #6:
Apple–Kiwi–Blackberry

Total Fat 1.4g

Saturated Fat 0.3g

Polyunsaturated Fat 0.8g

Monounsaturated Fat 0.1g

Cholesterol 0.0mg

Sodium 47.9mg

Potassium 901.9mg

Total Carbohydrate 99.4g

Dietary Fiber 18.2g

Sugars 52.9g

Protein 2.4g

Vitamin A 10.8%

Vitamin B12 20.0%

Vitamin B6 14.9%

Vitamin C 225.3%

Vitamin D 0.0%

Vitamin E 14.6%

Calcium 9.0%

Copper 23.0%

Folate 22.9%

Iron 9.5%

Magnesium 17.6%

Manganese 99.2%

Niacin 6.3%

Pantothenic Acid 5.2%

Phosphorus 8.7%

Riboflavin 8.3%

Selenium 3.1%

Thiamin 7.2%

Zinc 4.3%

Recipe #7:
Apple–Lemon–Ginger

Claimed to be "FOR: Joint pain"

Total Fat 0.9g

Saturated Fat 0.4g

Polyunsaturated Fat 0.4g

Monounsaturated Fat 0.0g

Cholesterol 0.0mg

Sodium 2.8mg

Potassium 607.2mg

Total Carbohydrate 72.6g

Dietary Fiber 15.3g

Sugars 41.4g

Protein 1.7g

Vitamin A 4.8%

Vitamin B12 20.0%

Vitamin B6 14.7%

Vitamin C 147.4%

Vitamin D 0.0%

Vitamin E 6.7%

Calcium 8.1%

Copper 19.9%

Folate 3.0%

Iron 7.6%

Magnesium 8.1%

Manganese 9.6%

Niacin 2.6%

Pantothenic Acid 4.6%

Phosphorus 4.3%

Riboflavin 5.4%

Selenium 1.7%

Thiamin 7.5%

Zinc 1.6%

Recipe #8:
Apple–Orange–Pear–Lemon

Claimed to be "FOR: Pain Reliever"

Total Fat 1.3g	Vitamin D 0.0%
Saturated Fat 0.3g	Vitamin E 10.1%
Polyunsaturated Fat 0.4g	Calcium 9.1%
Monounsaturated Fat 0.1g	Copper 18.2%
Cholesterol 0.0mg	Folate 14.7%
Sodium 0.0mg	Iron 5.9%
Potassium 762.1mg	Magnesium 9.3%
Total Carbohydrate 82.7g	Manganese 14.2%
Dietary Fiber 14.6g	Niacin 3.8%
Sugars 40.0g	Pantothenic Acid 6.2%
Protein 2.3g	Phosphorus 5.6%
Vitamin A 8.9%	Riboflavin 9.3%
Vitamin B12 20.0%	Selenium 4.4%
Vitamin B6 12.0%	Thiamin 12.9%
Vitamin C 153.5%	Zinc 2.6%

Recipe #9:
Apple–Raspberry–Orange–Spirulina

Total Fat 2.5g

Saturated Fat 0.8g

Polyunsaturated Fat 1.6g

Monounsaturated Fat 0.2g

Cholesterol 0.0mg

Sodium 6.2mg

Potassium 1,267.5mg

Total Carbohydrate 116.8g

Dietary Fiber 29.1g

Sugars 68.8g

Protein 4.8g

Vitamin A 19.0%

Vitamin B-12 0.0%

Vitamin B-6 35.5%

Vitamin C 300.4%

Vitamin D 0.0%

Vitamin E 22.3%

Calcium 16.0%

Copper 31.8%

Folate 30.8%

Iron 15.7%

Magnesium 22.5%

Manganese 141.5%

Niacin 18.6%

Pantothenic Acid 11.9%

Phosphorus 10.8%

Riboflavin 28.7%

Selenium 5.3%

Thiamin 34.6%

Zinc 9.8%

Recipe #10:
Apple–Strawberry–Banana

Total Fat 1.4g

Saturated Fat 0.5g

Polyunsaturated Fat 0.5g

Monounsaturated Fat 0.2g

Cholesterol 0.0mg

Sodium 1.9mg

Potassium 911.0mg

Total Carbohydrate 75.2g

Dietary Fiber 12.1g

Sugars 46.2g

Protein 2.1g

Vitamin A 5.1%

Vitamin B12 20.0%

Vitamin B6 43.0%

Vitamin C 116.0%

Vitamin D 0.0%

Vitamin E 6.6%

Calcium 3.7%

Copper 13.8%

Folate 10.9%

Iron 6.5%

Magnesium 14.1%

Manganese 26.2%

Niacin 5.1%

Pantothenic Acid 7.4%

Phosphorus 5.8%

Riboflavin 12.2%

Selenium 3.6%

Thiamin 7.6%

Zinc 2.6%

Recipe #11:
Blackberry–Raspberry–Strawberry

Total Fat 1.4g

Saturated Fat 0.5g

Polyunsaturated Fat 0.5g

Monounsaturated Fat 0.2g

Cholesterol 0.0mg

Sodium 1.9mg

Potassium 911.0mg

Total Carbohydrate 75.2g

Dietary Fiber 12.1g

Sugars 46.2g

Protein 2.1g

Vitamin A 5.1%

Vitamin B12 20.0%

Vitamin B6 43.0%

Vitamin C 116.0%

Vitamin D 0.0%

Vitamin E 6.6%

Calcium 3.7%

Copper 13.8%

Folate 10.9%

Iron 6.5%

Magnesium 14.1%

Manganese 26.2%

Niacin 5.1%

Pantothenic Acid 7.4%

Phosphorus 5.8%

Riboflavin 12.2%

Selenium 3.6%

Thiamin 7.6%

Zinc 2.6%

Recipe #12:
Blueberry–Blackberry–Strawberry–Grape–Lemon

Claimed to be "FOR: Healing Asthma"

Total Fat 1.7g	Vitamin D 0.0%
Saturated Fat 0.0g	Vitamin E 17.9%
Polyunsaturated Fat 0.2g	Calcium 14.4%
Monounsaturated Fat 0.3g	Copper 33.4%
Cholesterol 0.0mg	Folate 29.8%
Sodium 11.0mg	Iron 14.2%
Potassium 891.3mg	Magnesium 19.6%
Total Carbohydrate 68.2g	Manganese 216.8%
Dietary Fiber 23.3g	Niacin 9.8%
Sugars 38.8g	Pantothenic Acid 12.0%
Protein 4.1g	Phosphorus 9.7%
Vitamin A 13.2%	Riboflavin 15.2%
Vitamin B12 0.0%	Selenium 4.3%
Vitamin B6 16.1%	Thiamin 13.2%
Vitamin C 269.5%	Zinc 7.3%

Recipe #13:
Blueberry–Kiwi

Claimed to be "FOR: Immune System Strength, Younger Looking Skin"

Total Fat 0.9g	Vitamin D 0.0%
Saturated Fat 0.0g	Vitamin E 48.6%
Polyunsaturated Fat 0.6g	Calcium 10.5%
Monounsaturated Fat 0.0g	Copper 40.0%
Cholesterol 0.0mg	Folate 32.6%
Sodium 54.9mg	Iron 12.1%
Potassium 1,402.49mg	Magnesium 26.1%
Total Carbohydrate 136.4g	Manganese 102.0%
Dietary Fiber 27.3g	Niacin 18.7%
Sugars 75.0g	Pantothenic Acid 6.5%
Protein 7.4g	Phosphorus 16.5%
Vitamin A 22.6%	Riboflavin 28.1%
Vitamin B12 0.0%	Selenium 8.1%
Vitamin B6 23.2%	Thiamin 26.0%
Vitamin C 529.3%	Zinc 8.2%

Oran Kangas

Recipe #14:
Currant–Pineapple

Claimed to be "FOR: Easing PMS Symptoms"

Total Fat 2.2g	Vitamin D 0.0%
Saturated Fat 0.0g	Vitamin E 1.6%
Polyunsaturated Fat 0.4g	Calcium 125.4%
Monounsaturated Fat 0.2g	Copper 17.1%
Cholesterol 0.0mg	Folate 8.6%
Sodium 11.2mg	Iron 6.4%
Potassium 1,072.0mg	Magnesium 10.8%
Total Carbohydrate 72.8g	Manganese 255.6%
Dietary Fiber 3.8g	Niacin 6.6%
Sugars 32.0g	Pantothenic Acid 5.0%
Protein 4.4g	Phosphorus 2.2%
Vitamin A 1.4%	Riboflavin 6.6%
Vitamin B12 20.0%	Selenium 2.6%
Vitamin B6 13.3%	Thiamin 19.0%
Vitamin C 79.6%	Zinc 1.6%

Recipe #15:
Grapefruit–Papaya

Claimed to be "FOR: Healing Candida"

Total Fat 1.1g

Saturated Fat 0.3g

Polyunsaturated Fat 0.2g

Monounsaturated Fat 0.3g

Cholesterol 0.0mg

Sodium 18.2mg

Potassium 1,875.0mg

Total Carbohydrate 78.1g

Dietary Fiber 13.7g

Sugars 35.9g

Protein 5.1g

Vitamin A 145.8%

Vitamin B12 20.0%

Vitamin B6 10.9%

Vitamin C 777.9%

Vitamin D 0.0%

Vitamin E 36.9%

Calcium 18.3%

Copper 10.3%

Folate 63.3%

Iron 5.0%

Magnesium 20.1%

Manganese 4.6%

Niacin 12.7%

Pantothenic Acid 20.2%

Phosphorus 5.3%

Riboflavin 14.3%

Selenium 10.1%

Thiamin 17.5%

Zinc 4.0%

Recipe #16:
Melon–Apple–Pear–Lemon

Claimed to be "FOR: Boost of Energy, Cancer Prevention"

Total Fat 1.4g	Vitamin D 0.0%
Saturated Fat 0.4g	Vitamin E 8.2%
Polyunsaturated Fat 0.6g	Calcium 10.1%
Monounsaturated Fat 0.0g	Copper 22.7%
Cholesterol 0.0mg	Folate 25.7%
Sodium 92.5mg	Iron 10.9%
Potassium 1,579.3mg	Magnesium 18.6%
Total Carbohydrate 96.6g	Manganese 13.0%
Dietary Fiber 15.5g	Niacin 12.4%
Sugars 68.2g	Pantothenic Acid 11.5%
Protein 4.1g	Phosphorus 8.7%
Vitamin A 8.4%	Riboflavin 7.8%
Vitamin B12 20.0%	Selenium 6.1%
Vitamin B6 33.2%	Thiamin 18.6%
Vitamin C 284.1%	Zinc 4.2%

Recipe #17:
Orange–Apple–Raspberry–Strawberry

Total Fat 1.2g

Saturated Fat 0.2g

Polyunsaturated Fat 0.6g

Monounsaturated Fat 0.1g

Cholesterol 0.0mg

Sodium 0.8mg

Potassium 774.3mg

Total Carbohydrate 70.1g

Dietary Fiber 16.6g

Sugars 44.0g

Protein 2.7g

Vitamin A 10.3%

Vitamin B12 20.0%

Vitamin B6 14.5%

Vitamin C 239.9%

Vitamin D 0.0%

Vitamin E 7.9%

Calcium 9.6%

Copper 12.9%

Folate 19.2%

Iron 7.1%

Magnesium 11.5%

Manganese 50.0%

Niacin 6.5%

Pantothenic Acid 9.1%

Phosphorus 6.0%

Riboflavin 11.6%

Selenium 3.3%

Thiamin 13.0%

Zinc 3.8%

Recipe #18:
Orange–Carrot–Cinnamon

Total Fat 0.7g

Saturated Fat 0.1g

Polyunsaturated Fat 0.2g

Monounsaturated Fat 0.0g

Cholesterol 0.0mg

Sodium 126.3mg

Potassium 1,059.8mg

Total Carbohydrate 48.4g

Dietary Fiber 11.4g

Sugars 33.1g

Protein 4.2g

Vitamin A 451.3%

Vitamin B12 20.0%

Vitamin B6 20.5%

Vitamin C 250.3%

Vitamin D 0.0%

Vitamin E 7.3%

Calcium 16.5%

Copper 10.1%

Folate 28.3%

Iron 4.5%

Magnesium 12.0%

Manganese 16.5%

Niacin 12.6%

Pantothenic Acid 11.5%

Phosphorus 10.0%

Riboflavin 12.4%

Selenium 2.2%

Thiamin 23.2%

Zinc 4.1%

Recipe #19:
Orange–Grapefruit–Lemon

Total Fat 0.5g

Saturated Fat 0.0g

Polyunsaturated Fat 0.1g

Monounsaturated Fat 0.0g

Cholesterol 0.0mg

Sodium 0.8mg

Potassium 1,065.7mg

Total Carbohydrate 69.1g

Dietary Fiber 14.4g

Sugars 53.9g

Protein 5.5g

Vitamin A 24.9%

Vitamin B12 20.0%

Vitamin B6 18.4%

Vitamin C 537.4%

Vitamin D 0.0%

Vitamin E 6.8%

Calcium 23.4%

Copper 16.9%

Folate 40.6%

Iron 4.3%

Magnesium 15.2%

Manganese 7.1%

Niacin 8.1%

Pantothenic Acid 15.6%

Phosphorus 8.2%

Riboflavin 13.8%

Selenium 4.8%

Thiamin 33.0%

Zinc 2.9%

Recipe #20:
Pineapple–Grape–Ginger

Claimed to be "FOR: immune system, cold, cough, sore throat"

Total Fat 3.9g	Vitamin D 0.0%
Saturated Fat 0.6g	Vitamin E 13.6%
Polyunsaturated Fat 1.2g	Calcium 7.2%
Monounsaturated Fat 0.3g	Copper 41.0%
Cholesterol 0.0mg	Folate 16.2%
Sodium 21.2mg	Iron 14.4%
Potassium 886.7mg	Magnesium 21.2%
Total Carbohydrate 111.5g	Manganese 393.0%
Dietary Fiber 7.3g	Niacin 14.8%
Sugars 78.0g	Pantothenic Acid 8.3%
Protein 2.8g	Phosphorus 7.6%
Vitamin A 6.7%	Riboflavin 20.6%
Vitamin B12 20.0%	Selenium 4.9%
Vitamin B6 37.8%	Thiamin 48.2%
Vitamin C 177.2%	Zinc 5.1%

Recipe #21:
Pineapple–Orange–Grape–Strawberry

Claimed to be "FOR: Colds and the Flu"

Total Fat 2.9g	Vitamin D 0.0%
Saturated Fat 0.3g	Vitamin E 9.5%
Polyunsaturated Fat 0.9g	Calcium 10.7%
Monounsaturated Fat 0.3g	Copper 29.9%
Cholesterol 0.0mg	Folate 24.9%
Sodium 7.5mg	Iron 11.7%
Potassium 942.8mg	Magnesium 19.2%
Total Carbohydrate 77.4g	Manganese 277.5%
Dietary Fiber 10.2g	Niacin 12.0%
Sugars 65.1g	Pantothenic Acid 12.4%
Protein 3.6g	Phosphorus 8.2%
Vitamin A 9.7%	Riboflavin 19.2%
Vitamin B12 20.0%	Selenium 5.1%
Vitamin B6 29.2%	Thiamin 37.9%
Vitamin C 326.6%	Zinc 3.6%

Recipe #22:
Pineapple–Orange–Lime

Claimed to be "FOR: Lower Blood Pressure"

Total Fat 1.3g	Vitamin D 0.0%
Saturated Fat 0.0g	Vitamin E 3.1%
Polyunsaturated Fat 0.3g	Calcium 7.7%
Monounsaturated Fat 0.2g	Copper 17.5%
Cholesterol 0.0mg	Folate 17.2%
Sodium 3.0mg	Iron 6.6%
Potassium 542.4mg	Magnesium 12.4%
Total Carbohydrate 48.8g	Manganese 209.6%
Dietary Fiber 6.8g	Niacin 7.4%
Sugars 38.7g	Pantothenic Acid 7.8%
Protein 2.4g	Phosphorus 4.0%
Vitamin A 6.7%	Riboflavin 8.7%
Vitamin B12 20.0%	Selenium 3.2%
Vitamin B6 15.2%	Thiamin 23.5%
Vitamin C 190.6%	Zinc 2.0%

Recipe #23:
Pineapple–Papaya–Kiwi

Claimed to be "FOR: Ulcers"

Total Fat 2.7g	Vitamin D 0.0%
Saturated Fat 0.0g	Vitamin E 10.8%
Polyunsaturated Fat 1.0g	Calcium 7.3%
Monounsaturated Fat 0.3g	Copper 37.5%
Cholesterol 0.0mg	Folate 27.3%
Sodium 12.4mg	Iron 13.0%
Potassium 1030.2mg	Magnesium 27.6%
Total Carbohydrate 80.2g	Manganese 384.8%
Dietary Fiber 10.9g	Niacin 13.7%
Sugars 48.0g	Pantothenic Acid 7.5%
Protein 3.4g	Phosphorus 9.3%
Vitamin A 7.5%	Riboflavin 14.3%
Vitamin B12 0.0%	Selenium 5.3%
Vitamin B6 26.9%	Thiamin 30.5%
Vitamin C 367.6%	Zinc 4.2%

Recipe #24:
Plum–Orange–Ginger

Claimed to be "FOR: Anti-Aging"

Total Fat 2.5g	Vitamin D 0.0%
Saturated Fat 0.0g	Vitamin E 25.5%
Polyunsaturated Fat 0.0g	Calcium 10.0%
Monounsaturated Fat 1.2g	Copper 26.0%
Cholesterol 0.0mg	Folate 19.5%
Sodium 0.3mg	Iron 8.0%
Potassium 1,488.6mg	Magnesium 17.9%
Total Carbohydrate 105.8g	Manganese 22.3%
Dietary Fiber 13.9g	Niacin 18.7%
Sugars 90.4g	Pantothenic Acid 14.1%
Protein 7.2g	Phosphorus 15.1%
Vitamin A 60.6%	Riboflavin 15.1%
Vitamin B12 0.0%	Selenium 0.0%
Vitamin B6 16.1%	Thiamin 22.0%
Vitamin C 242.4%	Zinc 5.4%

Recipe #25:
Strawberry–Blueberry–Raspberry

Total Fat 1.3g

Saturated Fat 0.0g

Polyunsaturated Fat 0.7g

Monounsaturated Fat 0.2g

Cholesterol 0.0mg

Sodium 10.2mg

Potassium 568.4mg

Total Carbohydrate 45.4g

Dietary Fiber 15.8g

Sugars 23.0g

Protein 3.0g

Vitamin A 6.9%

Vitamin B12 20.0%

Vitamin B6 10.6%

Vitamin C 226.2%

Vitamin D 0.0%

Vitamin E 11.0%

Calcium 5.7%

Copper 12.7%

Folate 17.0%

Iron 8.5%

Magnesium 11.1%

Manganese 104.6%

Niacin 9.8%

Pantothenic Acid 9.5%

Phosphorus 5.9%

Riboflavin 16.7%

Selenium 3.8%

Thiamin 9.1%

Zinc 6.2%

Recipe #26:
Watermelon–Honeydew–Cantaloupe

Claimed to be "FOR: Lung Health"

Total Fat 13.4g	Vitamin D 0.0%
Saturated Fat 2.2g	Vitamin E 27.9%
Polyunsaturated Fat 4.2g	Calcium 29.8%
Monounsaturated Fat 3.0g	Copper 59.8%
Cholesterol 0.0mg	Folate 82.8%
Sodium 275.7mg	Iron 38.4%
Potassium 6,605.8mg	Magnesium 101.3%
Total Carbohydrate 300.6g	Manganese 67.2%
Dietary Fiber 24.3g	Niacin 59.1%
Sugars 273.5g	Pantothenic Acid 71.7%
Protein 25.3g	Phosphorus 41.2%
Vitamin A 532.0%	Riboflavin 40.1%
Vitamin B12 0.0%	Selenium 16.1%
Vitamin B6 237.2%	Thiamin 159.0%
Vitamin C 1,049.3%	Zinc 22.3%

Recipe #27:
Watermelon–Lemon

Total Fat 5.5g

Saturated Fat 0.8g

Polyunsaturated Fat 1.6g

Monounsaturated Fat 1.5g

Cholesterol 0.0mg

Sodium 26.2mg

Potassium 1466.7mg

Total Carbohydrate 93.4g

Dietary Fiber 11.1g

Sugars 74.3g

Protein 8.7g

Vitamin A 83.6%

Vitamin B-12 0.0%

Vitamin B-6 86.7%

Vitamin C 319.1%

Vitamin D 0.0%

Vitamin E 8.2%

Calcium 15.5%

Copper 32.1%

Folate 6.0%

Iron 15.4%

Magnesium 33.7%

Manganese 20.3%

Niacin 12.2%

Pantothenic Acid 27.0%

Phosphorus 12.0%

Riboflavin 15.6%

Selenium 1.5%

Thiamin 63.9%

Zinc 5.9%

Recipe #28:
Watermelon–Orange–Mango–Pineapple–Strawberry

Claimed to be "FOR: Healthy hair, clear eyes, and healthy skin"

Total Fat 3.8g	Vitamin D 0.0%
Saturated Fat 0.5g	Vitamin E 15.7%
Polyunsaturated Fat 1.0g	Calcium 12.3%
Monounsaturated Fat 1.0g	Copper 26.2%
Cholesterol 0.0mg	Folate 21.1%
Sodium 16.6mg	Iron 9.6%
Potassium 1,292.0mg	Magnesium 26.2%
Total Carbohydrate 97.6g	Manganese 78.8%
Dietary Fiber 10.3g	Niacin 14.4%
Sugars 85.2g	Pantothenic Acid 20.4%
Protein 6.4g	Phosphorus 9.8%
Vitamin A 76.2%	Riboflavin 17.5%
Vitamin B12 20.0%	Selenium 3.8%
Vitamin B6 62.0%	Thiamin 51.3%
Vitamin C 310.8%	Zinc 4.2%

Recipe #29:
Watermelon–Orange–Pineapple– Lemon

Claimed to be "FOR: Strengthener"

Total Fat 13.1g	Vitamin D 0.0%
Saturated Fat 1.6g	Vitamin E 27.3%
Polyunsaturated Fat 3.5g	Calcium 58.3%
Monounsaturated Fat 3.2g	Copper 85.8%
Cholesterol 0.0mg	Folate 79.6%
Sodium 53.1mg	Iron 37.6%
Potassium 4,583.4mg	Magnesium 95.4%
Total Carbohydrate 308.1g	Manganese 307.0%
Dietary Fiber 39.7g	Niacin 41.1%
Sugars 256.8g	Pantothenic Acid 76.8%
Protein 25.0g	Phosphorus 35.8%
Vitamin A 203.0%	Riboflavin 54.5%
Vitamin B12 20.0%	Selenium 11.3%
Vitamin B6 206.4%	Thiamin 190.2%
Vitamin C 1,280.9%	Zinc 16.3%

Recipe #30:
Watermelon–Pineapple–Orange–Kiwi–Lemon

Claimed to be "FOR: Strengthener"

Total Fat 13.5g	Vitamin D 0.0%
Saturated Fat 1.6g	Vitamin E 32.7%
Polyunsaturated Fat 3.9g	Calcium 51.8%
Monounsaturated Fat 3.3g	Copper 91.7%
Cholesterol 0.0mg	Folate 74.4%
Sodium 60.7mg	Iron 39.6%
Potassium 4,613.9mg	Magnesium 100.3%
Total Carbohydrate 299.9g	Manganese 303.6%
Dietary Fiber 38.6g	Niacin 41.3%
Sugars 232.0g	Pantothenic Acid 70.2%
Protein 24.0g	Phosphorus 38.3%
Vitamin A 197.5%	Riboflavin 52.8%
Vitamin B-12 0.0%	Selenium 10.7%
Vitamin B-6 205.4%	Thiamin 177.1%
Vitamin C 1,296.9%	Zinc 16.9%

Oran Kangas

PART 4: RESOURCES

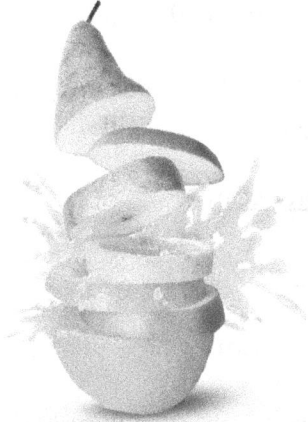

Intro

Winding down now.

Websites to investigate.

Potential hazards.

The huge and hugely informative glossary.

And we end with how to contact your humble author, aka me.

8: Websites Of Interest To Juicers

The FDA website has 2 excellent charts which summarize nutrition facts for fruits and vegetables:

http://www.fda.gov/Food/IngredientsPackagingLabeling/LabelingNutrition/ucm063367.htm

http://all-about-juicing.com

http://bestofjuicing.com

http://blog.jaykordich.com

http://ehow.com/search.html?s=juicing&skin=corporate&t=all

http://happyjuicer.com

http://healingfeast.com

http://healthy-juicing.com

http://juicing-for-health.com

http://myjuicecleanse.com

http://smoothiefactory.com

http://www.squidoo.com/juicingforhealth

http://thekitchn.com

http://worldwidehealth.com

9: Potential Hazards To Juicers?

Hazards in juicing? Are you kidding me? Well I guess with everything there is risk, but you'll feel better knowing that the Lancet, a very conservative medical journal, assures us that supervised *fasting* is extremely safe.

And juicing is a far safer process than fasting.

There, I feel better already, don't you?

Who Shouldn't Juice?

WARNING: Just to be safe you should consult your physician before you embark on a fabulous juicing journey. Not that juicing itself is dangerous, but you might have some underlying condition that requires immediate medical treatment. Besides, seeing a doctor would make my lawyer happy.

Now let's get crackin'.

Rumors say that the following groups shouldn't juice:

- Pregnant Women.
- Diabetics.
- Cancer Patients.
- People With Low Blood Pressure.

Truths are what we need, not rumors. Let's examine these special situations, case by case.

Pregnant Women

A pregnant body is utilizing HUGE amounts of vitamins and minerals to support a living being and to me it makes sense TO juice for this reason. But, as with everything, you need to use your noggin.

ANYTHING to the extreme isn't good, so things like parsley juice should be avoided because it can be toxic in large amounts.

Mommy ... Good. Fetus ... Maybe Not.

Of course the growing baby needs lots of vitamins and minerals, but *perhaps* it can't handle some components in huge amounts.

Also there is an idea of an addictive sort of process which *might* occur. That theory goes like this. The fetus grows accustomed to huge amounts of nutrients, so after birth will have a difficult time to maintain that level.

It's all theory there. So I advise caution.

Moderation would be crucial, if you choose to juice during pregnancy.

(Hold it, my attorney just advised me to refer you to your doctor, again. Well, if you think your doctor knows the answer to THIS question, when scientific researchers don't, you just go right ahead and ask her.)

Moving on.

Diabetics

The issue here is sharp spikes in blood sugar levels, not in the nutrition that juicing provides.

Simply put, it's best to go for the veggies and back off on the fruits a little. That is because fruits contain more sugars, the very ingredient that causes said spikes for said folks.

A moderate level of juicing that focuses upon low glycemic index carbohydrates (aka veggies) is perfectly safe. Indeed is quite healthy.

Fruits are not off-limits, they merely must be consumed slowly. Control the flow and away you go.

But go carefully and always listen to your body.

Cancer Patients

Maybe they are deemed too weak to handle the positive changes?

Start slowly and ease your way in. Juicing is especially beneficial for patients who aren't able to eat a lot. Like during chemo.

Your doctor's opinion might actually be of value here, as he knows the composition of the poisons he is intentionally putting into your body, admittedly for good reason. To kill cancer cells.

Just be aware that many people who have survived cancer have attributed their recovery to juicing.

I say, your body, your call.

People With Low Blood Pressure

I have extremely low blood pressure. So low that it makes my doctor does a double check every time that annual exam comes around. And I have absolutely no issues with juicing. It has only been a positive for me and my body's functioning.

This low BP myth is based on the fasting stereotype. People with low blood pressure shouldn't starve themselves to death. And for the record, no one else should either.

Juicing is not equal to water fasting. Eat sensibly and juice sensibly. Understood?

Other Special Situations

Finally let's look at controversial subjects that *might* apply to any juicer.

- Vitamin Deficiencies.

- Low Calcium?

- Fiber.

- Soy.

- Odds And Ends.

Vitamin Deficiencies

Some people believe that prolonged juicing is going to lead to serious vitamin deficiencies.

They're right! It could.

But only if you are really dumb in your juicing.

Fruits and vegetables actually have a lot more protein and fiber than you think and in the right combinations. So by SMART JUICING, you will do just fine.

You can always add high protein ingredients to your juice, like artichoke, asparagus, broccoli, Brussels sprouts, cauliflower, spinach or watercress.

Another perfectly acceptable solution is to occasionally add protein powder to your juice. It actually improves some flavors.

Low Calcium

Just up the broccoli or have a cool refreshing glass of milk.

Fiber

Fiber has many positive factors. We talked about some earlier. Here are more:

- Keeps blood sugar steady.
- Helps you feel full.
- Reduces risk of heart disease.
- Keeps food moving full-speed ahead through your body.
- Reduces risks of certain cancers.

Your body will tell you how much fiber you need.

Warning: It is in your best interest to add fiber *slowly* to your diet.

I should clarify the difference between soluble and insoluble fiber. So that's what I'm going to do without getting too 'sciencey' (my word) on you.

Soluble Fiber:

- Breaks down in water forming a jello-like substance.
- Helps moderate your mood swings from blood sugar fluctuations.
- Lowers bad cholesterol.

Some great foods high in soluble fiber are:

- Oatmeal, oat bran, nuts and seeds.
- Dry beans and peas.
- Strawberries and blueberries.
- Pears and apples.

Insoluble Fiber:

- Goes through your digestive system and pretty much stays intact.
- Reduces the risk of colorectal cancer, constipation and hemorrhoids.

Some awesome foods with insoluble fiber are:

- Whole wheat breads and cereals.
- Brown rice and seeds.
- Most vegetables and fruits.

Prune juice fits into our conversation here because it is an excellent natural laxative.

As I have stated **many** times throughout this book, fiber is good for you. My quick summary of the "battle" between fiber and juicing is that both sides are right; both are healthy choices.

Fiber and juicing are not natural enemies, they are best viewed as allies ... in the war against sickness and disease.

Soy

With many health benefits, soy is generally well regarded.

"Several large population studies have shown that consumption of soy foods is associated with a reduction in prostate cancer risk in men, is significantly associated with decreased risk of death and recurrence of breast cancer among women and may reduce the risk of colorectal cancer in postmenopausal women." Wikipedia.com.

"Recent studies have shown improvement in cognitive function, particularly verbal memory and in frontal lobe function with the use of soy supplements." Wikipedia.com.

However, the same source also notes that: "Allergy to soy is common."

More worrisome are conflicting studies on breast cancer in women: some find soy to be beneficial, others the opposite. A 2011 literature analysis concluded soy reduced rates in Asians, but not in Westerners.

Concerned people should do their own research to choose a path they are comfortable with.

Juicing really is for everyone, except maybe for the unborn.

Just be smart and watch what you drink.

A quick request: Amazon's advertising help for authors is heavily influenced by Customer Reviews. If you would take a couple of minutes to leave one, I would really appreciate it.

To leave a review, please go to http://amzn.to/1eeUlgG

10: Extraordinarily Comprehensive Glossary

(AKA Ingredients Of The Ingredients)

Remember that Glossary I told you about, way back in Chapter 1? In case you did not heed my advice and ingest the information in small, easily assimilated doses, like a juice, now you are face to face with a huge feast of scientific knowledge.

Well, better late than never. I'll let you get to it without further distractions. Then we'll chat afterward. OK?

1. Amino Acids

General Data

Amino acids are the basic units used in the creation of proteins. They join together in chains to form peptides or polypeptides (poly=many). The peptides link together creating proteins.

20 different types of amino acids can join up to create proteins, the specific type of amino acids dictate the resulting shape of the proteins formed.

The over-all structure of an amino acid molecule will include: an amine group, a carboxyl group, and a side chain. 1 carbon, 2 oxygen, and 1 hydrogen atom comprise the carboxyl group. An amine group, 1 nitrogen and 2 hydrogen atoms.

The 20 amino acids differ in the shapes, configuration, and molecule of their side chains.

Specifically, a protein is an amino acid chain, and an amino acid is simply a tiny molecule that has been assigned the role of a component to a cell. While carbohydrates give the cell the raw power it needs to perform, amino acids give the cell the materials it needs to build a big and strong body.

Amino acids are synthesized within the body from the food we eat.

In general, the human body is about 20% protein, 60% water, and the rest consists mainly of minerals, for example the calcium in bones. In nature there are about 100 amino acids, but your body uses only 20.

However, thousands of different proteins are necessary in your body. But don't worry: as long as you supply the 20 "building kits," your body can manufacture all those other proteins.

Now getting down to the nitty-gritty. There are 2 groupings of amino acids, labeled essential and non-essential. The so called non-essential amino acids are those which your body cleverly creates out of various chemicals in its internal storage system.

Dietary protein is obtained from either animal or plant sources; 'best' is the animal source, which is called a 'complete protein'. Which simply means it contains all the essential amino acids - no assembly required.

On the other hand, vegetable sources are not complete, they are missing some of these amino acids. Those are referred to as the "essential" amino acids. Meaning it is essential that they be created in order to function properly. OK, so far?

An example is rice, which is low in lysine and isoleucine. By combining specific vegetables, like a puzzle, you can create a perfect protein source. You just need to learn what goes with what. Welcome to the world of the vegetarian.

By using vegetable sources with lots of inherent proteins, you have the best shot at completing the amino acid puzzle. Beans with nuts and soybeans are one such successful combination.

Your digestive system is the engine that breaks down incoming proteins into their original amino acids, just before they are sent on their various missions through the blood stream.

Amino acids are literally the building blocks of life.

While carbs are critically important, don't think your body can survive on carbs alone. Your body can't make it without a steady supply of protein. But don't worry, there's about 8 grams of protein in a glass of milk and up to 3 grams in a slice of whole grain bread.

Beneficial Effects

The 11 Non-Essential Amino Acids (your body makes them):

Alanine – comes from pyruvic acid.

Arginine – created from glutamic acid.

Asparagine – derived from aspartic acid.

Aspartic Acid.

Cysteine – occurs in keratins and other proteins.

Glutamic Acid – created from oxoglutaric acid.

Glutamine – created from glutamic acid.

Glycine – made from threonine and serine.

Proline – derived from glutamic acid.

Serine – created from glucose.

Tryosine – made from phenylalanine (for neurotransmitters).

The 9 Essential Amino Acids (these must come from food):

Isoleucine – for muscle structure.

Histidine – essential component in the diet of vertebrates.

Leucine – a hydrophilic. For muscle structure.

Lysine – also important in diet of vertebrates.

Methionine – sulfur containing.

Phenylalanine – widely distributed in plant proteins.

Threonine – hydrophilic.

Tryptophan – essential vertebrate nutrient. Regulates sleep cycle, lowers anxiety, reduces depression, lowers artery spasm risk, strengthens immune system. For neurotransmitters.

Valine – constituent of most amino proteins. For muscle structure.

Vegetarians need to pay attention to their dietary proteins. Plant proteins are all missing at least 1 of the 9 essential amino acids. But not to worry, every amino acid has a plant form. You just need to combine the right plants to get all of the proteins you need.

2. Anthocyanins

General Data

Think red wine and no, more is not better. Anthocyanins help fight wrinkling of the skin and other inevitable aging consequences.

Beneficial Effects

Anthocyanins are thought to be a key ingredient in the heart-healthy properties raved about in red wine.

They promotes artery health:

1. Protect artery walls from oxidizing damage caused by free radicals (see below).

2. Help build and defend strong arteries.

3. Assist in keeping arteries elastic, which helps deter arteriosclerosis from developing.

They also help literally hold us together by aiding Vitamin C in the construction of collagen. That is the sticky firming substance that glues us together.

Good Examples

Brightly colored fruits, vegetables and flowers. The bright red in apples, deep purple in eggplant and blackberries, the bright red in blood oranges, the purple-leaf color of the European Beech and, of course, the deep red in red grapes.

3. Antioxidants

General Data

Large amounts of antioxidants are found in raw fruits and vegetables and various plant products. Vitamins C and E remove potentially damaging oxidizing agents in a living organism.

Sensibly, items with the highest concentrations of antioxidants offer the best protection against the damage caused by free radicals and some of the best antioxidant juices are made of 100% natural fruits and/or vegetables.

In general, the darker the color of an item, the greater is its concentration of antioxidants. Antioxidant fight free-radicals, by stopping the oxidation process in the body.

Beneficial Effects

Antioxidants help to prevent cancer, reduce the risk for atherosclerosis, lower blood pressure and protect the heart.

Components/Examples

Vitamins A, C, E, and a diverse range of plant components referred to as phytochemicals (see their own section below).

4. Carbohydrates (Carbs)

General Data

The primary energy source for your entire body, carbs come from plants. You eat the plants and your body extracts what it needs. You can use carbs right away, because of their quick energy production. Otherwise, your body converts them into body fat for later use.

You will find 3 kinds of carbs - sugars, starches, and fiber. Regardless their size, all carbohydrates are made from just 3 elements: carbon, hydrogen, and oxygen.

A simple sugar molecule (glucose) consists of 6 carbon atoms, 12 hydrogen atoms and 6 oxygen atoms (with a formula of C6(H2O)6) in the shape of a hexagon. This is what our brains and bodies depend upon daily for their energy.

Monosaccharide means "single sugar." Included in this group are:

- Glucose.
- Fructose – from fruits and veggies.
- Galactose – derived from milk.
- Ribose – is a component in ribonucleic acid (genetic transcription material).

Disaccharide means "2 sugars." Only glucose, fructose and galactose can create them. Types include:

- Lactose (milk sugar) comes from glucose and galactose molecules. "lactose-intolerant" refers to an inability to digest this sugar correctly.
- Sucrose (ordinary sugar) is composed of glucose and fructose molecules.
- Maltose (malt sugar) is created by processing cereal products, like barley.

Simple sugars are simple to digest. Glucose and fructose rapidly enter the blood stream through the small intestine. This is a problem for diabetics or those with metabolic syndrome.

Many tiny sugar molecules can come together to form a long chain, creating a large starch molecule known as a complex carbohydrate. This group includes:

- Starch, the energy storage unit for carbohydrates in plants. Starchy foods are: potatoes, wheat, corn, rice and carrots. They require special digestive enzymes to break down.
- Glycogen, energy storage unit for glucose in animals.

Your body does not process carbs from animal sources.

- Cellulose, the plants' structural element, which provides their shape like the skeleton does for us. Although we cannot digest cellulose, it is a key component of fiber, lignin, pectin, chitin, inulin, beta-glucan, and oligosaccharides. All are important to our health.

Dietary cellulose and starch are essential complex carbohydrates for nutrition. Dry beans, potatoes, rice, grain, squash, corn, and peas are rich in starch. For non-starchy veggies: cauliflower, broccoli, lettuce, asparagus, and greens. They contain even more indigestible cellulose, and they have the benefit of less calories.

Metabolism:

Your body starts the process of breaking carbs down to monosaccharides immediately. Simple sugars start to dissolve inside your mouth. Your saliva contains the enzyme Oranlase, which breaks down starch into glucose as you chew.

Carb digestion moves to the small intestine, which finishes the job with more Oranlase. The resulting monosaccharides are then absorbed by the blood, where they are immediately used for energy, saved as glycogen within the muscles and liver, or converted to long-term storage as body fat.

Storage is controlled by insulin, which tells the body to keep additional sugar in the form of glycogen. Individuals with metabolic syndrome and diabetics can't produce sufficient insulin (or they aren't sensitive to insulin).

For normal daily activities the body prefers glucose as its primary fuel. Muscles need glucose for movement; organs (including the brain) need it to operate. Even though the body creates glucose (from the protein and fats you eat), it's recommended that half of all calories originate from healthy sources of carbohydrates, for example, fruits, whole grain products, and veggies. Definitely not from candy, sodas, and cookies.

5. Chlorophyll

General Data

Chlorophyll is a nutrient found in plants that produces a characteristic green juice. When introduced into the human body, it becomes hemin, the darker the green is in a plant, the greater the amount of chlorophyll.

It helps plants grow and mature, and if depleted there would be less oxygen on earth.

You may remember from biology class that chlorophyll is a molecule that soaks up the sunlight and uses that energy to create carbohydrates from water and carbon dioxide. The process is called photosynthesis and it is responsible for sustaining life in all plants.

We eat the 'green' plants to get our chlorophyll. A good and healthy example is wheat grass.

Chlorophyll is mainly composed of carbon and hydrogen. Yet it is similar in structure to blood (with the tiny exception that the main atom in chlorophyll is magnesium, while in blood it's iron).

Beneficial Effects

Chlorophyll helps to:

- Improve circulation.

- Rebuild blood cells.
- Produce red blood tissues.
- Purify blood.
- Create hemoglobin.
- Detoxify the body.
- Strengthen the body.
- Cleanse the liver.
- Eliminate mold and parasites (yummy).

6. Enzymes

General Data

Technically speaking, enzymes are biological catalysts that regulate various chemical reactions internally. They are proteins which are derived from amino acids. They are powerful, yet fragile and heating destroys their vital ability to speed up chemical reactions.

Your best bet is to quickly quaff your raw fruits and vegetables right after juicing them, so you can use the enzymes before they deteriorate.

Enzymes act as helpers for thousands of chemical reactions which take place in the body. They are critical for digestion, absorption of food, converting food into body tissue, and for making energy on a cellular level. They also aid in strengthening the immune system.

Fact is that enzymes are crucial for most metabolic activities in your body. And fresh juices win the gold medal in the enzyme Olympics. It's the 'freshness' factor that is critical here, since heating and time kill the enzymes.

Did you know that if you cook your food over 118 degrees Celsius, you will kill almost all the enzymes?

When you eat, these digestive enzymes are released from your saliva glands, sending instructions to your stomach and small intestine to get prepped for digestion.

But by the time you are 30, you have used up all your digestive enzymes. That's why people often need to take supplemental digestion enzymes.

Luckily your body produces enzymes naturally, although the parts must be replenished. That said, if your body has an inadequate amount of enzyme intake, it will use those stored in your organs, which will lower your metabolism.

So, if you eat cooked or processed foods, you will definitely need additional enzymes to function optimally. Juicing raw fruits and vegetables provides your body the best source of fresh enzymes.

Beneficial Effects

Enzymes help your body in many ways:

- Improve digestion, so all your food can be utilized to power your body.
- Help protect cells from damage by toxins in food, air and water.
- Increase your metabolic rate to help you burn fat and calories.
- Strengthen your immune system to fight off disease, given an ample supply of phytochemicals.

Components/Examples

Most enzymes are proteins. Most enzymes catalyze reactions without help, but some need a non-protein component (called a co-factor, an inorganic ion).

Enzymes are recognized by the reactions they cause. The 6 classes are:

1. Oxidoreductases.

2. Transferases.

3. Lyases.

4. Isomerases.

5. Ligases.

6. Hydrolase.

And that's about as far as we're going to go with the technical stuff on this one.

7. Essential Fatty Acids

General Data

Essential fatty acids are 'essential' because your body isn't equipped to make them, so you must get them from food. Without going into the minutia, there are 2 specialized fats: omega-3 and omega-6 fatty acids which are needed for the proper functioning of all the tissues within the human body.

Essential fatty acids are stored in numerous parts of your body, including nerve cells and the cellular membrane around all cells.

It's important to find good sources of your omega-3 and omega-6 fats daily and take them in the right amounts. These 2 items must be balanced for optimal health.

Being deficient will cause:

- Liver and kidney problems.
- Growth issues.
- Poor immune system.
- Depression.
- Skin problems, like itchiness.

Unfortunately, the average U.S. diet is heavy with omega-6's, due to processed oils and foods. Fixing this issue is a matter of lowering omega-6 **and** increasing omega-3 acids.

The proper balance in intake will help:

- Prevent atherosclerosis.
- Lower risk of heart disease and stroke.
- Relieve symptoms of menstrual pain.
- Help joint pain.
- Improve ulcerative colitis.

Omega-6 Data

Omega-6 fatty acids are abundant in:

- Leafy green vegetables.
- Nuts, seeds, and grains.
- Vegetable oils (like corn, soybean, safflower, sesame, cottonseed, and sunflower).

Omega-6 acids are adequate in most diets. If anything, we get too much. It's the 3's we need to worry about.

Omega-3 Data

It is particularly important that vegetarians include omega-3's daily.

Omega-3 fatty acids are found in:

- Hemp oil.
- Fish like salmon, herring, sardines, tuna, and halibut and algae.
- Vegetables and fruits.
- Beans, nuts and seeds.
- Flax seeds (best source).
- Canola (rapeseed).
- Soybean, wheat germ and walnuts.
- Soya products.
- Whole grains.

It's recommended that you eat fish a few times a week.

Omega-3 fatty acids are also referred to as polyunsaturated fatty acids. They are concentrated in the brain.

Symptoms of deficiencies are:

- Fatigue.
- Poor memory.
- Dry skin.
- Heart problems.
- Mood swings.
- Depression.
- Poor circulation.
- Unborn babies are at risk for eye and nerve problems.

Beneficial Effects

- Important for cognitive and behavioral functions.
- Child development.
- Reduce the risk of heart disease.
- Reduce inflammation.
- May lower the risk of cancer.
- Improve chronic diseases, like arthritis.

8. Flavonoids

General Data

Flavonoids are also referred to as Vitamin P, because of their effect on the permeability of vascular capillaries.

They are polyphenlic compounds which are everywhere in nature, categorized by their chemical structure: flavonols, flavones, flavonones, catechins, isoflavones, anthocyanidins and chalcomes.

Researchers have identified more than 4,000 unique types, mainly in beverages, fruits and vegetables.

Interestingly enough, flavonoid consumption is inversely related to death by coronary heart disease, as well as heart attack incidence. So drink up, so you can live it up.

The flavonoid contribution to the antioxidant defense system could well be substantial, especially considering a person's total daily intake ranges from 50 – 800 mg. This is extremely high, the average daily amount of other antioxidants, for instance Vitamin E is 7-10mg, C is 70mg, and carotenoids only 2-3mg.

Oxidation of LDL (low-density lipoprotein) plays a big role in atherosclerosis. What happens is immune system macrophages identify and surround oxidized LDL, which leads to atherosclerotic plaque on the walls of the arteries.

LDL oxidation is produced by the macrophages and it is helped by metal ions, such as copper. Numerous studies show flavonoids protect LDL from this oxidation.

Beneficial Effects

Flavonoids have recently aroused special interest because of their beneficial effects and reports that they have properties which are:

- Anti-allergic.
- Antiviral.
- Anti-Inflammatory.
- Anti-Platelet.
- Antioxidant.
- Anti-Tumor.

By contributing to the total antioxidant defense system, flavonoids help protect your body against:

- Cancer.
- Aging.
- Atherosclerosis.
- Ischemic injury.
- Inflammation.
- Neurodegenerative diseases (Parkinson's and Alzheimer's).

Examples

- Quercetin.
- Picatechin.

Great sources for flavonoids are:

- Citrus.
- Berries.
- Onions.
- Parsley.
- Tea.
- Red Wine.
- Dark Chocolate.

Did I hear a cheer there at the end? I guess it was just my imagination.

9. Free Radicals

General Data

Free radicals are simply unstable oxygen molecules that occur naturally in the body during metabolism; and are also found in UV light. Free radicals are found in polluted air, environmental contaminants, and natural oxidation. Due to increased global pollution, we need more antioxidants than ever.

The danger is that the toxic heavy metals located in our aquatic systems and seafood, act as poisonous free radicals when they set foot in our bodies. It's primarily the carotenes, which are plant pigments that help keep free radicals from damaging the body and help improve the immune system.

Carotenes in kale, spinach, chard, beet greens, watercress, mangoes, cantaloupe, broccoli, apricots, and romaine lettuce are a few of the unsung heroes.

Detrimental Effects

Free radicals are anything but helpful for your body. Here are some of their dangers:

- Can damage DNA.
- Lead to certain forms of cancer.
- Cause damage to the arteries, leading to impaired cells and inflamed artery walls.
- Lead to hardening of the arteries.
- Contribute to plaque buildup, leading to arteriosclerosis.
- Attack the nucleus of cells and cell walls. Damaged mutations can develop into cancer.
- Cause cardiovascular disease.
- Cause Alzheimer's disease.
- Cause Parkinson's disease.

Components

These are atoms, molecules or ions left with unpaired electrons. This is technically called an open shell configuration.

I just call them 'an open invitation to disaster.'

10. Minerals

General Data

Minerals are highly sensitive to heat and without this sensitivity we couldn't assimilate them into our bodies. Cooking basically destroys most valuable nutrients.

Although minerals are fairly resistant, they still get lost when cooked, because they diffuse into the water. Also plant nutrients come as a 'whole' and are dependent on each other.

Raw juices are the best way to preserve the holistic goodness of the vegetable.

Components/Examples

In order to gain a wide array of minerals you should juice:

Calcium: beet greens, broccoli, celery, carrots, dandelion greens, kale, parsley, oranges, romaine, string beans, spinach, watercress.

Iron: asparagus, beets with greens, blackberries, broccoli, cabbage, carrots, cauliflower, chard, parsley, dandelion greens, pineapple, strawberries.

Magnesium: beet greens, beets, blackberries, broccoli, carrots, cauliflower, celery, dandelion greens, garlic, parsley, spinach.

Manganese: beet greens, apples, beets, broccoli, cabbage, carrots, oranges, peaches, spinach, pears, tangerines.

Potassium: cabbage, asparagus, carrots, cauliflower, celery, chard, garlic, parsley, radishes, spinach, watercress.

Selenium: carrots, cabbage, chard, garlic, grapes, oranges, radishes, turnips.

Zinc: carrots, cabbage, cucumber, garlic, ginger root, grapes, parsley, spinach, tangerines, turnips.

Beneficial Effects

Minerals help improve:

- Eyesight, growth, appetite and taste (Vitamin A).
- Nervous system, digestion, muscles, and heart (Vitamin B1).
- Red blood manufacture and nerve formation (Vitamin B12).
- Immunity, viral protection, healing wounds, cholesterol, and cell lifespan (Vitamin C).

Numerous minerals are essential for correct functioning of the cells and tissues within the body, including:

- Aluminum.
- Calcium – bones and teeth.
- Chloride.
- Chromium.
- Cobalt.
- Copper.
- Fluoride.
- Iron.
- Magnesium.
- Manganese.
- Potassium.
- Selenium.
- Sodium.

- Sulfur.
- Trace minerals – only in small doses!
- Zinc.

11. Phytochemicals

General Data

Right now they are at the forefront of nutritional research. Although fairly new to the scene, more are being discovered all the time.

When they are at work, some phytochemicals bind to the cell walls to stop pathogens from entering. That is one reason they are considered by many to be the most powerful natural ingredients for fighting disease.

Researchers are excitedly focused on phytochemicals and substances that help construct or trigger enzymes, and their research is producing new discoveries continuously.

Beneficial Effects
- Antioxidants.
- Anti-inflammatory and anti-cancer properties.
- Hormonal action.
- Anti-microbial effects.
- Numerous amazing and diverse health benefits.

Components
- Indoles.
- Lutein and zeaxanthin (dark, leafy greens), slows age-

related macular degeneration.

- Lycopene is a potent anti-oxidant with anti-cancer properties, helps lower cholesterol.
- Omega-3 fatty acids.
- Phenolic acids.
- Phytosterols.
- Protease inhibitors.
- Saponins.
- Soflavones.
- Sulforaphane: broccoli, Brussels sprouts, cabbage are thought to inhibit tumor growth.

12. Proteins

General Data

Protein digestion starts with chewing and continues in the stomach with hydrochloric acid and pepsinogen. Pepsinogen becomes pepsin, which breaks down the amino acid bonds. Meanwhile, the stomach muscles squeeze foods and acids together.

When the results arrive at the small intestine, the hydrochloric acid is neutralized and the pancreas releases the enzyme trypsin. It finishes breaking the amino acids apart, which are swept into the blood stream and carried to waiting cells throughout the body. Once at their destination, the amino acids are reused to construct new proteins for their new function.

To build the structural elements of the human body, like organs and muscles, proteins are essential. They are also necessary to maintain the immune system, neurotransmitters, and hormones.

All the proteins you need for a healthy body are available in any balanced diet. Eggs, meat, and dairy products are good animal sources, and legumes, grains, seeds and nuts are fine plant sources.

Proteins are large molecules made from amino acids (see Amino Acids above).

There are many proteins within your body lending a figurative hand.

Beneficial Effects:

- Contributes to enzyme activity.
- Promotes chemical reactions.
- Signals to cells their needed activities.
- Transports substances through your body.
- Keeps ph and fluids balanced.
- Serves as hormone building blocks.
- Helps blood clotting.
- Promotes antibody activity for allergy and immune control.
- Gives shape to body parts.

13. Vitamins

General Data

Well juiced fruits and vegetables are an incredible source of vitamins and you can get all the vitamins you require in 1 shot.

Vitamin A is not in plants, but its precursor (beta-carotene) is in orange vegetables and fruits. It is converted into Vitamin A within the body.

B1 or thiamine is found in beans, lentils, nuts, milk, oats, oranges, rice, seeds, wheat, whole grain cereals and yeast. And foods that are high in inositol are: oranges, grapefruit, peaches, cantaloupe, strawberries, watermelon and tomatoes.

In order to get pantothenic acid, have a bowl of kale, cantaloupe or cauliflower. Some foods rich in Vitamin B3 include: peanuts, wheat bran and brewer's yeast. And you can find lots of B5 in peanuts, mushrooms, split peas, soy beans and soy flour and B6 in spinach, kale, turnip greens, bell peppers and prunes.

Tasty fuel rich in B12 vitamins includes: tempeh, tofu and foods high in folic acid, including: soy, white beans, Lima beans, chickpeas, lentils, spinach and cooked asparagus.

Folic acid is critical for pregnant woman early in pregnancy to help prevent developmental issues with the growing baby. Folic acid is found in sunflower seeds, romaine lettuce, peanuts and orange and pineapple juices.

Although there are numerous foods that provide B vitamins, juicing gives you the pure shot your body will best assimilate.

As for vitamins C, the body cannot make it and thus gets it from food. Fruits and vegetables are a great source, for example, citrus fruits and parsley, which has 3 times the amount of Vitamin C of oranges. Other awesome sources are: kale, broccoli, Brussels sprouts, watercress, cauliflower, cabbage, strawberries, papaya, spinach, turnips, mangoes, asparagus and cantaloupe.

Vitamin C is water soluble and readily absorbed.

Vitamin D is found in sunflower seeds, sunflower sprouts and mushrooms and good old sunshine is your best source, in moderation, with sunscreen, of course.

Juicing from Vitamin E enriched products gives your body the optimum dose of this important vitamin that it can take in at once. E is be found in spinach, watercress, asparagus, carrots, tomatoes, blackberries and kiwi. It is an oil soluble vitamin.

Beneficial Effects

Vitamin A:

- Helps ensure good eyesight.
- Critical for proper functioning of the retina.
- Prevents night blindness.
- Reduces the risk of age-related cataracts and macular degeneration.
- Antioxidants prevent cellular damage that can trigger cancer.

Vitamin B:

- Repairs and renews tissues.
- Critical for energy.
- Keeps skin, muscles and organs healthy.
- B6 and b9 aid in the formation of proteins that make red blood cells.

Vitamin C:

- Essential in creating collagen, the glue that holds you together.
- Helps maintain healthy gums and capillaries.
- Promotes iron absorption.
- Helps repair skin cells.

- Creates a healthy immune system.
- Builds quality blood supply.
- Antioxidants prevent cellular damage that can trigger cancer.
- Reduces depression.
- Creates an acidic environment to prevent painful urinary tract infection.
- Reduces the risk of age-related macular degeneration and cataracts.

Vitamin E:

- Helps prostate health.
- Prevents oxidation in the metabolism of fat.
- Protects the cells from dangerous free radicals.
- Helps prevent plaque in the blood vessels, which can lead to stroke and heart disease.

Vitamin C, E and B complex vitamins are all necessary for the body to remain strong and resilient, yet often the modern diet is deficient in these vitamins because of the large amount of processed foods we ingest.

ONWARD, to juicing, health, and eternal happiness!

Or you can just go back to the office on Monday morning.

11: Conclusion

You've done it! You've learned:

- The benefits of juicing.
- How to do it.
- 30 great fruit, melon and berry juicing recipes.
- A healthy lifestyle.

I hope that you enjoyed this book. And that you continue to juice your way to good health.

If you have suggestions for future changes to this book, please let me know. Contact information is on the last page.

You can do me a big favor, if you're in a favoring-doing sort of mood. Amazon's advertising aid to authors is heavily influenced by Customer Reviews. If you would take a couple of minutes to leave one, I would really appreciate it.

To leave a review, please go to http://amzn.to/1eeUlgG

Copyright & Legal Notices

About The Author: Oran Kangas

Oran is a researcher specializing in health and healing. He is also an avid, long-time juicer. Now in his 70's, he attributes his good health to the healthy practice of daily juicing.

He attended college for so many years that he considered himself a professional student.

"Eventually I stumbled out into the real world. Armed only with 2 Master's degrees, I soon realized that a marketable skill would have been a smarter choice. I scurried back to college. Computers were the new bright shiny object that held my attention ... for the next half century."

Even today Oran spends 12 hours a day, 7 days a week staring at the 1-eyed beast that stares irrevocably back.

His true calling came shortly after finally leaving college – the martial arts. With black belts in Kung Fu and JuJitsu, lesser rankings in Judo, Aikido, and TaeKwanDo, and the traditional non-ranking of Tai Chi, he was ready to take on the world, figuratively and literally.

He settled into a life of teaching. But Life had other plans for the teacher. In his mid-30s his body gave out. With no other choice, he closed down his school and opened up a search: to learn the name of his hidden assailant. 10 years later there was a name (several, actually), but no cure (and there still isn't). It was an auto-immune dysfunction – his body had betrayed him at the cellular level.

With no body to depend on, our intrepid Author-To-Be returned to the world of the mind. The computer was his labor-saving tool and education, in the form of research, his career. His primary target: health.

After many false starts, he heard of juicing, and immediately saw it as the next step in nutrition-based health.

He now lives in Northern California with his wife and a herd of cats.

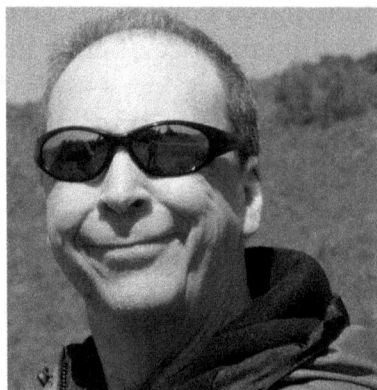

Contact Page

Connect With Me Online:

- **Website:** BigIdeas-Publishing.com
- **Email:** okangas@BigIdeas-Publishing.com

Other Books By Me:

Productivity: Big Ideas From The Top 10 Books

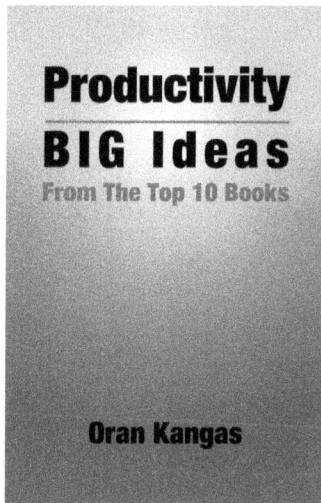

Kindle Edition - http://amazon.com/dp/B00BQH98O0

Paperback Edition - http://amazon.com/dp/1484069765

Recommended Reading:

Note: The following are NOT affiliate links. I have no financial interests or agreements with these (competing) authors. Trust me, someone always worries about such matters. 1 critic knocked me down 2 stars on the above book based on a suspicion that I received a fee – not true, but what can I do?

- **The Juicing Bible** by Pat Crocker
  http://amazon.com/dp/0778801810

- **The Big Book of Juices** by Natalie Savona
  http://amazon.com/dp/1844839737

- **The Everything Juicing Book** by Carole Jacobs, Chef Patrice Johnson & Nicole Cormier
  http://amazon.com/dp/B0046H9KN6

www.ingramcontent.com/pod-product-compliance
Lightning Source LLC
Chambersburg PA
CBHW050114280326
41933CB00010B/1094